"The intriguing complexi[...] a deadly disease, its extraordinary resilience against treatment, its attacks on the immune system, and its interplay with aging—are unveiled before the reader's eyes while being immersed in Dr. Weeraratna's life stories. She takes us on a captivating journey through what shaped her as a person and as a scientist, revealing how each step in her career added a new piece to the puzzle of her research."

—Margaret Foti, PhD, MD (hc),
CEO, American Association for Cancer Research

"This is storytelling at its best. The journey of the author's upbringing and how her experience with myriad cultures has informed Dr. Weeraratna's work in the pursuit of understanding and defeating cancer as we know it is fascinating. Her story is particularly inspiring for anyone who might be interested in pursuing a career in STEM."

—Sung Poblete, PhD, RN, CEO of Stand Up To Cancer

"Dr. Weeraratna's amalgam of her personal history, her lab's cutting-edge research on the increasingly important link between cancer and aging, and the promise, hopes, and limitations of future anti-cancer therapies is a beautifully accessible account for scientific and nonscientific audiences alike."

—Judith Campisi, PhD, Professor, Buck Institute for Research on Aging;
Senior Scientist, Lawrence Berkeley National Laboratory

"This clear and optimistic insider's view on how cancers form and become aggressive, and what's being done to alter their courses toward remissions and recovery, is a captivating read for anyone whose life has been touched by the disease. Dr. Weeraratna—an acclaimed researcher on age-related differences in how people respond to certain cancer treatments as well as a fierce advocate for junior faculty, women, immigrants, and people of color in science—presents the human side of medical lab work and will inspire budding future scientists from underrepresented backgrounds and other countries."

"Dr. Weeraratna's research at the vanguard of aging's impacts on metastases and treatments, and her remarkable journeys as an immigrant scientist and advocate, inform this clear, fascinating narrative of both the nature of cancer and advancements in the campaigns against it, providing us with evidence-informed hope from her own and others' labs that we're actually beginning to curb the destruction of this horrible disease."

Is Cancer Inevitable?

JOHNS HOPKINS
WAVELENGTHS

In classrooms, field stations, and laboratories in Baltimore and around the world, the Bloomberg Distinguished Professors of Johns Hopkins University are opening the boundaries of our understanding on many of the world's most complex challenges. The Johns Hopkins Wavelengths series brings readers inside their stories, presenting the pioneering discoveries and innovations that benefit people in their neighborhoods and across the globe in artificial intelligence, cancer research, food systems, health equity, science diplomacy, and other critical areas of study. Through these compelling narratives, their insights will spark conversations from dorm rooms to dining rooms to boardrooms.

This print and digital media program is a partnership between the Johns Hopkins University Press and the University's Office of Research. Team members include:

Consultant Editor: Tim Wendel

Senior Acquisitions Editor: Matthew R. McAdam

Copyeditor: Charles Dibble

Art Director: Martha Sewall

Series Designer: Matthew Cole

Production Designer: Bea Jackson

Production Supervisor: Jennifer Paulson

Program Manager: Anna Marlis Burgard

JHUP Director and Publisher: Barbara Kline Pope

Office of Research Executive Director for Research: Julie Messersmith

Is Cancer Inevitable?

ASHANI T. WEERARATNA, PhD

with Tim Wendel

Johns Hopkins University Press
Baltimore

Johns Hopkins Wavelengths is a trademark of the Johns Hopkins University

© 2021 Johns Hopkins University Press
All rights reserved. Published 2021
Printed in the United States of America on acid-free paper
9 8 7 6 5 4 3 2 1

Johns Hopkins University Press
2715 North Charles Street
Baltimore, Maryland 21218-4363
www.press.jhu.edu

Library of Congress Cataloging-in-Publication Data

Names: Weeraratna, Ashani T., 1970– author. | Wendel, Tim, author.
Title: Is cancer inevitable? / Ashani T. Weeraratna, PhD., with Tim Wendel
Description: Baltimore : Johns Hopkins University Press, 2021. | Series:
  Johns Hopkins wavelengths | Includes bibliographical references and
  index.
Identifiers: LCCN 2021018587 | ISBN 9781421442747 (paperback) | ISBN
  9781421442761 (ebook open access) | ISBN 9781421442754 (ebook)
Subjects: LCSH: Cancer—Age factors. | Cancer—Research. | Carcinogenesis.
  | Older people—Diseases.
Classification: LCC RC261 .W415 2021 | DDC 362.19699/40072—dc23
LC record available at https://lccn.loc.gov/2021018587

A catalog record for this book is available from the British Library.

Special discounts are available for bulk purchases of this book. For more information,
please contact Special Sales at specialsales@jh.edu.

Contents

Preface

I'LL NEVER FORGET THE FIRST TIME I looked through a microscope. I was immediately enthralled by how single-celled organisms in a microcosm can move around, replicate, and interact with each other. That first glimpse when I was 11 ignited a lifetime of curiosity. It's led me to tackle many of the questions I'm striving to answer today: What are the signaling pathways that drive a cancer cell to change its shape, replicate, or move from one site in the body to another? How does it communicate with the cells around it? A cancer cell is not an island—it doesn't exist or grow in isolation—so how does it interact with surrounding tissues, bone, and blood? Why does aging impact both the likelihood of a diagnosis and its mortality rate?

Cancer's resiliency can be remarkable. For example, if you give a normal cell a drug or treatment, it will respond in a predictable manner. But give a cancer cell something that's supposed to stop it, and more often than not it says, "Oh, this is a problem," and then takes extraordinary measures to repel whatever obstacle it encounters in order to keep moving ahead.

Through the work in my laboratory at Johns Hopkins University and in others around the world, we researchers are gaining better understandings about this formidable foe in many of its hundreds of forms. Building on the work of pioneering scientists who came before us, we're pushing toward better treatments and better outcomes. We have more clues now as to why healthy cells become cancerous and better understandings about the genetic materials present when we're conceived that can become activated as cancer cells many years later. Following cancer's trail is rarely a linear pathway. At times, it reminds me of how I found the path to study biology and to work in this field. My life story and my cancer research are often intertwined.

During the last decade or so, I've focused my research on revealing how changes that occur as we grow older can alter cancer cells, making them more aggressive—and learning why we become more susceptible to them in our advancing years, specifically as witnessed in melanoma tumor growth. My biggest motivation is the patients, first and foremost. A sobering 1,806,590 Americans were estimated to be diagnosed with a form of cancer in 2020, with more than 600,000 expected to die from it, according to the American Cancer Society,[1] while 17 million worldwide receive the terrifying news from their doctors, according to the World Cancer Research Fund.[2] Cancer isn't like other diseases. With diabetes, for example, you can exercise to maintain a healthy weight, watch your diet, and take insulin shots to live a normal life. But cancer remains a stubborn disease that we're still trying to fully comprehend, let alone control. It still leaves us helpless in many ways. I hate the unfairness of it, and I want to help turn the tide for these patients, their families, and the health care providers who work so hard to save them.

A WORLD AWAY

My fighting spirit and sense of justice have their roots in my childhood. My family left Sri Lanka when I was 2 years old, during the beginnings of what would become a civil war between the Sinhalese government and the Tamil Tigers, a terrorist guerrilla organization that arose in response to discriminatory policies against the Tamil people.

It used to be that when colonized countries gained their independence, most who knew how to run the basic operating systems—water supply, electric grid, transportation infrastructure—returned home, leaving those systems to fall apart because few of the indigenous people had been trained to take over. This is part of what gave the impression that these newly freed countries couldn't survive without their colonial rulers, further feeding the narrative that the colonized countries were somehow "primitive" and thereby ignoring their rich cultures and capabilities.

My dad's job was to work in collaboration with organizations like the United States Agency for International Development and the Canadian International Development

Agency to help train the Sri Lankan people to run these systems. Gerald William Weeraratna had a law degree, but he acted more like a diplomat in these times and situations. He helped smooth out that difficult transition from the outgoing colonists to the newly independent countries, teaching the people there how to manage these new systems. His favorite saying was "Give a man a fish, he will eat for a day. Teach a man to fish, he will eat for a lifetime." (I still have a handcrafted award given to him, of a hand holding a fish with those words inscribed.) I admired him—and now identify with him—so much, because what he was doing sometimes bordered on the impossible, or so it seemed to me, his second daughter and youngest child. He also taught me the importance of my voice, often asking my advice—even when I was only 10 years old!—on the phrasing of the questions for tests he prepared, on current politics, and even on his math.

Dad moved us to Africa in 1972, when I was a toddler. We went first to Zambia, in Central Africa, and lived there for four years before moving on to Lesotho in 1976. That's mainly where I grew up. Lesotho, a tiny country about the size of Rhode Island, known for its stunning snow-capped mountains and jaw-dropping waterfalls, gained its independence from Great Britain in 1966. Completely surrounded by South Africa, it's one of only three landlocked independent nations, along with Vatican City and San Marino. We lived in the capital city of Maseru in a lovely rancher that had a large yard leading to sprawling orchards of apple and peach trees. I used to hide in the branches of a massive willow and read books, totally undisturbed.

South Africa had more resources than Lesotho, and so for anything "extra" we wanted to do, we had to drive ten minutes to cross the border, which had checkpoints and guards. We crossed to go to the mall and for my ballet lessons, among many other reasons. Sometimes it was a fast crossing; we had a pass that made things easier. But other times the wait could last for hours, especially if the guards were in a bad mood and took their time questioning someone in a car ahead of us. It was an unusual and often frustrating way to live, but my childhood in Lesotho was formative in positive ways, too.

Most countries needed some kind of representation with South Africa but were reluctant to put an embassy or officials there because of the negative optics associated with the apartheid government. So, many of these countries had their embassies in Lesotho instead. As a result, the school that I went to, Machabeng College, had four hundred students, but they represented more than seventy nationalities. I feel so fortunate to have grown up with this incredibly diverse population, surrounded and nourished by all those languages, customs, and ways of looking at the world—an experience I've continued in my professional life by working with many other immigrants and people from across the United States.

Growing up where I did, amid such diversity, I had a lot of

advantages that I wouldn't trade for the world. But it was also a period of tremendous upheaval and turmoil, especially in the 1980s, during the last vicious throes of apartheid. As teenagers surrounded by South Africa, we took to the streets to protest the regime's injustices—I still have a small scar on my chin from a policeman's rifle butt. A course at our school encouraged our participation in civil protest. All of it made me less afraid to stand up for what's right, whether it's for more diversity in the STEM disciplines (science, technology, engineering and mathematics) or making sure that junior faculty have access to the resources that they need. Growing up in such a place, during such times, made me a conscientious but also stubborn person. Only my husband can tell you just how stubborn sometimes! That's something of which I'm strangely proud.

Around this time, my sister, Sharmila, used to drive me to school. At one point I had a science project growing cultures of dirt and grass in a petri dish; I watched the microcosm evolve over time and studied the growth of microbes daily under the microscope. The cultures smelled simply awful, like miniature swamps. Sharmila called them my "festering hay cultures." To this day, she'll say with great affection, "So, what's going on? How are your festering hay cultures?" Our private joke is a reminder to me that you have to put in the work, even when things are a little tedious, and kind of stink, because the answers are in there. There are no days off when you're working against cancer. Whatever form it may take, whether it's dormant or racing ahead, it's usually trying to outwit you. You have to stay on top of everything going on in your own lab, even the labs of others whose work could influence your outcomes.

Some might compare discovering ways to combat cancer to superheroes battling the bad guys. It's true that there's a need to be constantly vigilant and resourceful against the wily, dangerous enemy. Am I waging battles against cancer on a daily basis? Maybe, but they're often methodical and are won in increments, sample by sample, and data set by data set. But what keeps me going, what has intrigued me for decades now, is how resilient cancer can be. The ways that it can move and "talk" and change constantly remind me how imaginative we need to be in dealing with this disease in all its many forms. We have to respect this opponent.

For example, if you came face to face with an attacker and you were able to shoot him, you'd think that would be the end of it, right? But what if he somehow healed that bullet wound and stood up again? That's impossible, right? Or say another attacker could magically put his hand over a knife wound to heal it—mend himself so well that he was able to keep on going. Sounds like a superpower a character in a graphic novel might have, doesn't it? Yet that's the way cancer often works. That's the very nature, even the power, of how a cancer cell can transform itself. It fights back.

Such resiliency means we need to think about cancer much differently than we would about other chronic diseases, such as heart disease or diabetes. With those, we can give someone a bypass or a stent or drugs. Those procedures can prolong a life by years, or even decades. We may someday reach similar measures with cancer—longer remissions and, someday, outright cures, are the goal.

Cancer differs from other diseases in what measures we can take to control it because cancer is much more unpredictable and resistant. What I find remarkable is that it only takes a few cells for cancer to proliferate. That's a key difference between cancer and heart disease—between cancer and other illnesses. If only a few cancer cells somehow escape treatment or detection, they can cause major problems later on as they continue to replicate into tumors and split off and travel to other parts of the body.

We're finding now that tumors can leave a primary site very, very early in their life history, before they're even detected, and go to distant sites and just remain there, waiting. It's called tumor dormancy, one of cancer's most disturbing proclivities. And then, as we age, changes in the body drive those tumors out of dormancy and make them grow and metastasize. For example, with melanoma, we can take a biopsy from a 30-year-old who may have early signs of cancer. At this point, those cancer cells may not be that dangerous. But when that same patient is 65, additional changes could occur in those cells that could lead to metastatic melanoma in the lungs—it lies in wait.

TAKING A STAND

From my teenage days in Lesotho, having teachers who urged us to understand what was happening in the world and to act driven by conscience, I learned to be a fighter. The racial strife that has once again erupted in America has triggered some of those memories from my childhood in Africa. That kind of background, growing up in such times, has made me less tolerant of seeing people being treated unfairly. When Nelson Mandela was released from prison in 1990 after 27 years, I felt so joyous that I wasn't able to concentrate on anything for the rest of the day. I was in college halfway around the world at that point, but I knew his release was not just symbolic—it represented a sea change, one that had been a long time coming.

I had a philosophy class in high school titled the Theory of Knowledge. A quotation from that class that has stayed with me is Mahatma Gandhi's adage: "Be the change you want to see in the world." One of my favorite classes back then was community service. For that we did things like digging ditches to slow erosion and going to villages to help fit people for eyeglasses or administer vaccinations. Social justice and social work were activities that many of us in that class did together. We were proud to take up a social cause, to take a stand. These classes shaped my world view.

But while I look back on our time in Africa as my great adventure, there were minuses, too. If I saw a tin can on the road or a paper bag, I knew that I shouldn't kick it because there might be a bomb inside. I learned that if I saw a car parked alone on the side of the road, I should cross the road and not walk next to it, because it might have an even bigger bomb inside. I suppose it's similar to the United States, where kids know that if an alarm sounds in school, they need to huddle in a corner, sheltering in place because there might be a school shooter. Dangers arise in many places.

Years ago, I was in Edinburgh, Scotland, visiting my brother, Tino, and his family. It was my first visit there and we were walking around Edinburgh Castle, when the cannon went off, which it does every day at noon. I grabbed my niece and nephew, threw them to the ground and covered them with my body. It was instinctive. But my relatives were baffled, thinking, "What on earth are you doing?" It was my past coming back to life. Yet how does one fully explain something like that? How do those reactions become hardwired? In a way cancer cells are like that—programmed to survive and respond to their environment, and learning ways to adapt to it.

A FASCINATION WITH SCIENCE

Where I was in the family birth order must have had an effect, too. I'm the youngest of three kids. My brother and sister are much older—I'm the baby in the family by a good seven years. When we were living in Zambia, and my brother and sister reached high school age, my parents decided that the local schools there weren't strong enough. In that way, my parents were typical South Asian parents: education was the only thing that mattered to them. So, my brother and sister were sent to boarding school in the United Kingdom. For a time, they were like cousins who came to visit during the summer holidays. It was hard, because I was very attached to them, and particularly idolized my big brother, Tino, with whom I've always had a special relationship. Four-year-old me would always pack a bag for myself (books, a night dress, toothbrush, and snacks) to accompany him to the airport, hoping against hope that somehow, this time, they'd let me on the plane with him. To this day, my siblings and I are extremely close, even though we are continents apart.

Being on my own while they were away at school taught me the importance of being independent. Even now, though I work with amazing people in my lab and I'm surrounded by a loving family, I'm comfortable being on my own. I didn't mind being an only child much of the time, pretty much left to my own devices. Eventually, my brother moved back to Africa with his wife for a time, and my sister moved back as well, and for a short period we were all together. This was when I was 13 and my sister often drove me back and forth to school. That's when we first discussed those "festering hay cultures."

My mother, Carmen Lorette Wickramasinghe, was a strong, independent woman. Her mother, Grace Tucker, was the product of European colonialism—half English and half Portuguese. Her father, Leslie Wickramasinghe, was an aristocratic man whose vice was playing billiards in his local country club. He died of cancer before I was born, as did my mother's only brother. As for my mother, I'm told that she was an absolute rascal growing up. All the boys were afraid of her because she had a gorgeous older sister, and Lorette would beat up any boy who gave her sister grief. She was captain of the neighborhood boys' rugby team when she was 16. Most girls of the 1950s gravitated toward more genteel sports.

Just two years later, at 18, my mother married my father and then gave birth to my brother a year later. Even though she wasn't expected to go on to college, she always valued education. Her uncles were world-renowned astrophysicists, one at the University of Oxford and the other at the University of California, San Diego. She came from an academically rich, scientifically oriented and accomplished environment, but back in the 1950s girls weren't expected to pursue much along those lines.

When I came along and proved to be a good student, Mom was all over that, making sure that I did my homework and helping me prepare for exams. She always told me, "You can do anything you want, but you need to stand on your own two feet. Never depend on a man. Never." She told me this even though she loved my father dearly. Still, she was of the mind that life, at least *my* life, was not just about getting married and having babies. "Your life is to go out there," she told me, "and do something big."

Like a lot of people who go into the sciences, my favorite class was biology. It has been my great love all my life. The subject became even more important to me after my favorite ballet teacher died of cancer. I had begun dancing when I was 3 and continued until I was 16. Sticking to the strict regimen of ballet taught me that when you really love something, putting that level of work into it can be a real joy. I was serious about it and was very close to my instructor, Carla De Bruyn, a white South African woman who came across the border to teach us. Despite growing up in a small town in South Africa, Carla had a class of every color of kid you can imagine, given the diversity in Lesotho. She wasn't afraid to dream big about what we could do.

I remember her arguing with my mum. At first, my mum thought the dancing was cute and good exercise for her chubby daughter. As I grew older, and spent three hours a day practicing, she told me I had to drop it, so I could focus on my studies. Anyone who's pursued an international baccalaureate in high school or had a child who's done it knows it isn't easy, and now I kind of see my mum's point. Yet Carla stood her ground in supporting me, too. In the end, she convinced my mum to drive me ninety minutes each way, three times a week, to go to a dance class across the border in South Africa. Carla had a higher-level class there, and she felt I was ready for it. As a mother now, I admire my mum's devotion to cultivating my interests, even for something she didn't agree with, simply because I loved it.

When Carla became ill and then died of colon cancer in her fifties, I was devastated and decided that I needed to know more about this disease that took her from us, along with my uncle and grandfather. Because Maseru was the capital, it had a British High Commission nearby, with a good library. Probably to my mother's relief, after Carla's death I became a regular visitor there. The librarian helped guide my interests by showing me TV specials about science, even though I was an audience of one.

My favorite was "Life on Earth," a BBC series. Presented by David Attenborough, the show went all around the world, detailing animal life including the mountain gorillas in Rwanda that Attenborough encountered in Dian Fossey's sanctuary. My favorite episode was about how whales feed. They make a huge circle and form a cylinder that fills with fish. That allows the other whales to come in and eat all the fish. I thought that was so cool. The show offered me a glimpse of the worlds that existed well outside our landlocked country. By watching those programs and going through that library of books, I began to dream about what I could see and even do in the bigger world that lay beyond the border we crossed every day.

I became a heavy reader. I spent hours in the library, and I eventually worked my way through its entire collection of encyclopedias, along with lots of *National Geographic* issues. My mum used to call me the "Encyclopedia Lesothania," instead of the "Encyclopedia Britannica," because I would recite endless bits of knowledge. Today, I'm still pretty good at Trivial Pursuit, though I'm not sure how well that's served me.

What that time in the library did was allow me to dream. Leafing through all those books, learning as much as I could about the world around me, and about the disease that took Carla so prematurely, eventually led to the idea of pursuing a career in cancer research. By the time I was 16, I had decided that I would run my own laboratory one day. And I knew that the best place for that, where the best work was happening, was the United States.

COMING TO AMERICA

Of course, it's a long way from Maseru, Lesotho, to St. Mary's College in southern Maryland, where I completed my undergraduate studies—8,139 miles to be exact. Even though my brother and sister had gone to school in the United Kingdom, I was adamant that I needed to go to college in the United States. At first, my parents wouldn't hear of it—they were absolutely horrified when I first brought it up. Their vision of America in the 1980s was that everyone was on drugs and carried guns. There was no way they were allowing their youngest child to go there alone. Still, I knew that the best medical cancer research was being done in this country. "That's where I'm going to go," I told them and dug in my heels, which led to one of the very few major fights I had with my father.

Despite their objections, I laid out all my arguments about how the best programs were in the United States, but my dad wanted me to go to Oxford or Cambridge. And on and on we argued. Still, I believe my parents, especially my father, were impressed by the research I had done about college—how I was clearly stating my case about a subject that was near and dear to both of them—education. My dad believed it was the great equalizer, that if he could educate everyone around him then they'd all have an equal shot at a good life. In my own way, I believe that, too. To become a fisherman, so to speak, I knew I had to go to America to pursue my studies.

Finally, Mum and Dad said I could go but that I needed to enroll at a college close to friends. We had family friends, the Sengamalays, in Washington, DC, and even though it can be a two-hour drive or longer in traffic to where I ended up, my parents agreed. Further complicating things was that I wasn't 18 yet, so those friends needed to become my guardians, too. Over the years they and their two boys have become my family here, and that means so much more than I can express.

So that's how I ended up attending college at a small, beautiful, completely rural campus of maybe fifteen hundred students located on a peninsula extending into the Chesapeake Bay—a far cry in every way from landlocked Lesotho. It helped that St. Mary's College had been so persistent in recruiting me. I had also applied to George Washington, Vassar, and Hamilton, but St. Mary's had so few international students that it needed more. They called and called, and my mum said, "Oh, they really care about you." As it turns out, they did. I'm still great friends with Rich Edgar, the admissions director at the time, and now the college's director of development. I lived with his beautiful family on their farm for a couple of months after graduating, and they joke that they still refer to their guest room as "Ashi's room." They also taught me how to use a vacuum cleaner, an Amish drill, and many other useful skills. Going to St. Mary's is one of the best decisions I ever made, and it proved to be an amazing experience. It was my first real step into a field in which I very much wanted to have a major role. One of the key things the college did was to arrange summer internships in laboratories; I worked at the University of Maryland in Baltimore and also at the university's Chesapeake Biological Laboratory on beautiful Solomons Island close to the college. Those internships were vital in cementing my interest in a research career.

That said, my experience was also shaped by being one of only a handful of kids of color on campus at the time. And I was a foreigner—no one else on campus had an accent like mine, and my classmates and teachers didn't really know what to make of me. I adapt very easily, but some of my classmates—maybe not so much. I found it more amusing than anything else when people would ask me, "Do you ride elephants to school in Africa?" At first, I'd try to educate them, but sometimes—I hate to admit it—I'd just make stuff up. "Of course, I ride an elephant to school back home," I told them. "In fact, I've got a few in the garage."

Other than that adjustment, and maybe, in part, because of it, St. Mary's was exactly the right place at the right time because it allowed me to be absorbed by American culture. Everyone was so warm and friendly and embracing. Still, I had no clue about American culture at all, especially as a young adult. I remember my first couple of days in college. All the girls would sit in the hallway outside of their rooms and they would talk, getting to know each other. I would be in my room thinking, "Oh, I really wish I could join them." I thought some-one had to invite me. That's how it would have been in my British-leaning culture, the way I was brought up. Finally, one of the girls saw me in the bathroom and asked, "How come you never sit in the hallway with us?" I didn't know it was that easy to join them.

Because I had graduated from high school with an inter-national baccalaureate, I went straight into upper-level biol-ogy classes at St. Mary's. There were some struggles early on. I hadn't taken many multiple-choice tests before coming to college, which really threw me. And I was docked points for using British instead of American spelling. My biggest disas-ter was flunking organic chemistry. That was the first course I had ever failed, and given how critical it is to a career in the sciences, it was a big setback to overcome. Yet, through it all, I loved my classes, especially those having to do with biology, and I graduated in three years. I knew I'd made the right choice in studying this field.

After graduating from St. Mary's in 1991, I came to Johns Hopkins for the first time, becoming a senior technician in the school's oncology center. My mentor there was Bob Casero. He took great care of all of us who worked for him, and through him I began to see the role I could play in medicine, that it would be a mixture of doing important research and being able to mentor and foster others—by running my own lab someday. The idea of running my own lab had been with me since high school, but at Johns Hopkins I began to envision how to make it a reality.

Still, I must have had one of the worst first days on the job ever at Hopkins. I had broken my foot when a horse, a Persian workhorse (from the Edgars's farm), which are simply huge, had stepped on it. So, I showed up on my very first day in a cast. And things went downhill from there.

We were looking at an experiment on a UV box. It had a dish of water, with mutagen in a solution for a project about DNA. You turn out all the lights, put on a plastic shield, and, turn on the UV box. So, I went into the darkroom with the director on the project, my other boss and mentor, Paul Celano. He said, "I'm going to turn off the light. You pick up the plastic shield and put it on your face." In the dark, I picked up what I thought was a plastic shield. I brought it up to my head, and it went "Splash!" It wasn't the shield at all. It was the container full of staining solution. As the lights came on, my boss saw me standing there—all wet. That's when I just dropped the now empty container all the way over my soaked head. He shook his head and said, "Probation period: three months."

Of course, the story is now legend, part of my origin story. When Bob Casero introduced me for my chair, my current position at Johns Hopkins, he said how proud he was of me, and how I had "learned new ways to image DNA" when I was in his lab.

Despite some missteps and mistakes along the way, I've always been comfortable in the lab. In many ways, it feels like a second home, where I should be. Many days I'm as excited by what I'm witnessing as I was at the age of 11, peering through that microscope for the first time.

When you're a woman, you sometimes receive conflicting messages about how far you should or can go in medicine. The messages might be something like, "Maybe you shouldn't go on to grad school. Stick with what's easier." Early in my career, someone told me I was more suited to be a technician, that I probably shouldn't pursue a PhD—it might be too difficult, too much, for someone "like me." Both a professor in college and a professor (at the time) in the very department I now chair told me not to bother with graduate school. Even later in my career, there were points where I was told I wouldn't be allowed to continue. Being a woman of color made it no easier—I often had to fight for everything from recognition for my ideas, to a seat at the table, to promotions and advancements. But in situations like that, my stubbornness is an asset, and I've always known in my heart that this is where I belong, even if it means that others not used to people who look like me aren't comfortable with it and need to overcome that to make space for me.

Thankfully, I had people around me who were giving me more positive messages, about how I could—how I should— keep going further. And, over time, that became an important part of my personal philosophy. What more could I do, especially when it came to understanding cancer?

This curiosity and fascination with the world, first glimpsed back in Lesotho, took me from my graduate studies at the George Washington University to Johns Hopkins, the National Institutes of Health, the National Institute of Aging, The Wistar Institute, and back to Johns Hopkins. What more can we learn, discover and, ultimately, accomplish when it comes to cancer? In recent years, we've made great strides, many of which I'll tell you about. Much has changed for the better in recent decades. Our research is branching off into what were unseen directions only a few years ago. When it comes to cancer, the level of cooperation and understanding is now worldwide—a true international effort.

Undoubtedly, what lies ahead won't be easy. But coming this far wasn't, either. Managing or controlling cancer? Making sure a diagnosis doesn't become a death sentence? For me, there's no more captivating or challenging task right now in medicine.

Is Cancer Inevitable?

CHAPTER 1

The Nature of Cancer

THE EARLIEST KNOWN MEDICAL RECORDS of cancer can be found in ancient Egyptian papyri (thought to date from 2500 BC sources) that were deciphered in the nineteenth century. The texts reference a procedure for cauterization of breast tumors along with pharmacological and magical treatments—and recognize the difference between benign and malignant growths.[1] From fourth-century China, Taoist and doctor Hong Ge's *Urgent Therapeutic Prescription for Axilla Diseases* describes breast tumors as carbuncle stones with roots that infiltrate surrounding tissue.[2] Ancient Greek physicians including Hippocrates, Galen, and Paul of Aegina, a seventh-century scholar who wrote about breast cancer in his *Medical Compoendium in Seven Books*, likened the spreading tentacles of a tumor from its central form, and its grip on surrounding flesh, to that of a crab, or *karkinoma*—the Latin term is *cancer*, which entered into other European languages. The work and translations of the tenth-century Islamic physician and philosopher Abu Bakr Muhammad ibn Zakariya al-Razi (Rhazes in Latin) introduced Greek, Syrian, Arab, and

Indian medical knowledge to a broader audience, including substantive narratives on the diagnosis and treatment of cancer. Among other contributions, he was one of the earliest scholars and practitioners to introduce the concept of chemotherapy by combining alchemical, chemical, medical, and pharmacological knowledge.[3]

In spite of its early history of study, cancer seemed to fade into the shadows of medical discussions for long periods of recorded history. Other deadly, typically infectious diseases—tuberculosis, smallpox, typhus, cholera, influenza, typhoid, malaria, measles, yellow fever, and the plague—became the more immediate concerns given their enormous death tolls.[4] Simply put, not enough people in previous eras lived long enough to develop cancers, let alone suffer and die from them, for the disease to be a primary research focus. In addition, before autopsies were commonly conducted and other modern detection approaches were invented, communities often didn't know what people died of if it wasn't outwardly apparent.

Centuries later, lifespans expanded, and inventions such as the microscope, and disciplines including more informed observation, were added to the study of cancer. For example, in 1775, the English surgeon Percivall Pott introduced the first understanding of carcinogenic environmental agents when he discovered a high incidence of scrotum cancer among a population of chimney sweeps.[5] In 1902, German zoologist

Theodor Boveri recognized the genetic basis of some cancers.[6] The 1926 breast cancer studies of English physician Janet Lane-Claypon laid the groundwork for the field of cancer epidemiology.[7] The list goes on; multitudes of researchers and practitioners have continued to investigate and report their findings in an effort to understand and defeat cancer's myriad manifestations, with advances in technology aiding their work and its dissemination.

Siddhartha Mukherjee, author of *The Emperor of All Maladies*, writes that doctors in the nineteenth century linked cancer to the rise in civilization, believing that it "was caused by the rush and whirl of modern life, which somehow incited pathological growth in the body. The link was correct, but the causality was not: civilization did not cause cancer, but by extending human life spans—civilization unveiled it."[8] During the last century, the average life expectancy increased from 47 years to 76 for men and 81 for women.[9] More than half of the adults age 85 in 2011 were expected to live another six years, according to the Federal Interagency Forum on Aging-Related Statistics. In addition, the population of Americans ages 85 years and older was projected to grow from 5.5 million to 19 million by the year 2050.[10] By that same year, more than a quarter of our population will be over the age of 50—part of the common worldwide trend. Melanoma, for instance, is a cancer that is particularly susceptible to the ravages of aging.[11]

Of course, with the advent of modern medical techniques

and procedures, it also became easier to detect cancer. Soon efforts were underway not only to learn more about this disease, but to try to control, even cure it. Yet cancer has proved to be an elusive adversary, a shapeshifter that continues to confound medical experts.

MANY DISEASES IN ONE

What makes cancer so difficult to control is that it comprises scores of diseases, not just one. The fundamental, unifying characteristic of cancer is the abnormal growth of cells. This process can begin almost anywhere in the body, and as the cancer cells start to multiply, they crowd out the normal cells, making it too difficult for the body to function properly.

Beyond growing more quickly than normal cells, cancer can also spread to other parts of the body. This is called metastasis, and the process makes it much more difficult to halt cancer. My laboratory at Johns Hopkins is working to understand what drives the aggressive nature of tumors, and what makes them spread around the body and learn to resist therapy. There are more than one hundred types of cancer, including skin cancer, lung cancer, prostate cancer, and leukemia. Among these are forms that kill millions of people while some subtypes are so rare that only a dozen cases are documented worldwide.

Chemotherapy, surgery, radiation, and immunotherapy

have had varying levels of success in slowing, and sometimes stopping, this growth of abnormal cells. But due to the wide range of cancers, a treatment effective against one form doesn't necessarily work that well on another. We've come to understand that there is no magic bullet. No treatment or vaccine has yet been found that can stop all cancers, and I don't believe that we'll find a single cure. I think that our next steps should be determining how to *modify* this disease, so that's where my focus is right now.

In recent years, our lab has investigated how important a patient's age can be when it comes to types of cancer to which they may be susceptible, and how dangerous that cancer will be for them. Treatments or medicines that work well with a younger patient, for example, might have little or no effect for a patient 55 or older. Such insights have led us to become more precise and specific with our approach and methodology.

With cancer, processes rarely happen in isolation. When a person receives an unfortunate diagnosis, it may seem like a bolt out of the blue: stunning and arbitrary. Yet the more secrets we unravel about cancer, regarding how it forms and moves and interacts with other parts of the body, the more we realize that cancer has intricate methods and complex languages of its own.

Of the 1.8 million annual new cancer cases in this country, more than 200,000 will be melanoma diagnoses, one of the few cancers whose incidence is rising significantly—by more than 44 percent in the last decade.[12] Unlike the very common basal cell and squamous cell carcinomas, melanoma is a highly aggressive form of skin cancer, with a survival rate of only 27 percent for late-stage cancers.

The skin is the largest organ in the body. According to *National Geographic* magazine, which published a landmark issue about skin in 2017, adults carry an average of 8 pounds (3.6 kilograms) and 22 square feet (2 square meters).[13] This packaging of ours is waterproof and provides insulation and protection from wide ranges in temperature and the damaging rays of the sun. Formally called the cutaneous system, skin is its thinnest on the eyelids and thickest on the heels of our hands and feet.

Some skin types are more likely to suffer from melanoma, including those that are more prone to burning than tanning after exposure to the sun. People who spend a lot of time outdoors, such as athletes and outside laborers, are more likely to develop skin cancer. One's vulnerability can also depend upon how rigorously such measures as the use of sunscreen and wearing rimmed hats were applied in childhood and adulthood.

The outer layer of our skin is called the epidermis. Home to the protein keratin, which is also found in nails and hair, the epidermis layer also contains Langerhans cells, which alert the body's immune system to infections and viruses. The epidermis connects with the dermis, our deeper skin layer. Fibers of collagen and elastin give skin its elasticity and strength. These break down as we age, resulting in wrinkles and making us more vulnerable to cancer. That's because one of the dermis's key tasks is to nourish the outer layer, the epidermis, with its network of blood and lymph vessels.

Melanocytes—cells with long protrusions that look rather like weird sea creatures—are found in the epidermis's lower region, near the boundary with the dermis. These cells produce melanin, the darker pigments that are a primary factor in skin coloring. When they're working well, in concert with other body components, the melanocytes direct pigment to cells in the upper layers of skin, providing a natural sunblock. People native to regions closer to the equator have adapted over time by producing more melanin particles. In comparison, those who originate from lands farther to the north or south are prone to be fairer in skin color—seemingly an effective adaptation until people shift more radically and quickly in location. For example, sunny Australia, where much of the population is of northern European descent, has among the world's highest rates of skin cancer.

The epidermis and dermis layers sit atop the extracellular matrix. It all fits together like a cake, as my graduate student Gloria Marino loves to describe it, perhaps because she is a superlative baker herself. You have the frosting (epidermis), the cake (dermis), and the cake stand (the extracellular matrix, or ECM).

In recent years, we've also learned that genetic or microenvironmental changes can trigger cancer movement, signaling it to move elsewhere in the body and start invading. At first, the melanocytes may begin to grow out of control in a particular spot. Left untreated, a single melanoma growth can work its way down from the epidermis layer and into the dermis layer, where it can grow larger. Once it does so, reaching this lower level in the skin, the cells have access to blood and lymph vessels—gateways to the rest of the body. Think of it as a car that was once restricted to traffic-clogged, two-lane streets. This melanoma car has hit the on-ramp to a high-speed freeway. It can now travel throughout the body and become a life-threatening illness.

The microenvironment is defined as the immediate, small-scale world of a cell or group of cells. Instead of looking at everything from on high, a satellite view so to speak, we've zoomed way in, looking at this particular world—the surfaces and tissue surrounding the cell. We can think of the microenvironment as the neighborhood where the tumor lives. And the other components, or "people," will make up this neighborhood.

In the microenvironment, it benefits the tumor to know the guy who lives in the house next door and who's down the street. As in any neighborhood, there are a lot of different types of houses and a lot of different types of residents. In this case, they are the other cells. In this context, the world of the microenvironment, the way the streets run, which direction they go, which ones are one-way, is critically important. Also, how the houses are constructed. How stable are they? How permeable? How big? All of this makes up the biophysical matrix of the cancer.

Just as important, we need to know how the "people" in this neighborhood, in this microenvironment, interact with the tumor—how they communicate with it. The initial conversations may be the equivalent of, "What's the best way to get to the grocery story?" In the case of cancer cells, that translates to finding the best places or host areas where they can grow.

At a higher level, these relationships can be about who's going to be a friend. Who's going to be their ally and help them grow and even move? Those are the kind of neighbors in the microenvironment the cancer will seek out. Ultimately, it has a profound influence on the cancer cells and what level of destruction they can achieve.

Once the cancer goes deeper, through that first layer in the epidermis and into the dermis, it reaches the fibroblasts, which act like the skin's construction workers, providing the collagen and elastin. They're the most common cells of connective tissue in animals. At this level, the signals going to that tumor cell can be many and of great consequence.

We know that like many other cancers, melanoma is a disease of aging. The incidence of melanoma increases dramatically after the age of 60, and the prognosis is worse for the elderly, who present with more metastatic disease and respond more poorly to most therapies. Part of why we see less metastasis in younger people is because of these conversations—you may have more signals to the cell telling it to stay where it is in younger people. In older people, you can have more signals telling the cell, "Hey, get out of there. Go find a better site and really colonize."

In the lab, we can use fibroblasts of different ages and by doing so change the overall age of the artificial skin we grow for our research, offering us great insights about the impact of tumor cell behavior, as well as the role of aging. (For more about how this skin is made, see pages 70-74.) Our studies show that the melanoma cells are more likely to invade other parts of the body in the elderly than in the young. That's because in younger skin, the epidermis and dermis layers are more defined. The skin in younger people is firmer, less wrinkled, which you would expect. Yet when you look closer, through the microscope, you see that the melanoma also stays in tight nests, right near the surface of the skin, in the younger skin. The makeup of the collagen is that much thicker in such cases.

In comparison, when we study the skin of those ages 55 to 65 everything can be much different. Here, the melanoma cells are able to move more easily. The skin isn't holding them in place as much. The skin has been worn down over time; that means the cancer could move to the subcutaneous tissue—the blood, the lymphatics. This makes it easier for the cancer to travel throughout the body.

When tumor cells are in a firm setting or matrix, they cannot move around that well. But put those tumor cells in the skin matrix of an older person and then they can start to swim. The cancer cells love those possibilities. It can be so liberating for them. What was once holding them in place has lost its firm grip upon them. The door has swung open, and they can now break off and travel to locales elsewhere in the body.

THE RISK FACTORS

The risk of melanoma is slightly higher if one of your first-degree relations (parents, brother, sister) has or had melanoma. About 10 percent of those with melanoma have a family history of the disease. Those who are fair-skinned and even freckled run a higher risk of the disease. Our biological parents provide the genetic blueprints for our bodies. Genes are long sequences of DNA that help make the necessary proteins for bodily functions. For example, such proteins determine our eye color, height, hair color, and muscle mass, among many other characteristics; they can be switched "on" or "off," determining whether specific characteristics are expressed or not.

To understand gene modification, we need to delve briefly into the structure of chromosomes. Strands of DNA are wound around proteins called histones, which can look like beads on a string, with the histones serving as the beads and the DNA as the string wrapped around them. When DNA is loosely packed, or the string is not tightly wound around the histone "beads," a DNA sequence can be read and used to produce proteins. In essence, the gene is switched on. But when the DNA is tightly packed, the physical trait associated with this gene will not be expressed, and the gene is switched off.

External stimuli, such as long-term exposure to the sun or other factors in our environment, can determine whether genes, including those connected to cancer, are activated or remain dormant. Genes are basically the codes of the body. They are what says to the cell, "you need to do X, Y, or Z." Whether it's time to grow; whether it's time to move. And to do that we need to make these proteins that are going to help us do these different things.

Once those genes are activated and the proteins made, pathways are downstream. Think of it as the genes being the instruction manual, while the pathways are the gears and the mechanics of how the cell is working. Normal cell growth or uncontrolled cell division depends upon what has been switched on or off.

While men and women suffer from melanoma at almost the same rate in the United States (that 60:40 ratio), women often survive longer. We aren't sure why, but hormones may be a key consideration. We're now trying to understand how cells in men and women age differently and how that contributes to tumor progression. It could also be that women take better care of themselves, in terms of prevention and visits to the dermatologist if something is seen as out of the ordinary.

The cell of origin in melanoma is the melanocyte. It's dotted with dark black pigment, known as melanin, which it can pass to other cells, specifically keratinocytes, to protect them from the sun. Weirdly, when these cells start to become cancerous, they start to look more like the normal epithelial cells you find in the precursors for other cancers. Once melanocytes become melanoma, they may take several different forms and appearances. Most common is *cutaneous melanoma*, on the skin. *Acral lentiginous melanoma* is found on the hands and soles of the feet. Reggae singer Bob Marley, for example, developed this form of melanoma in his big toe, which spread to his brain. *Mucosal melanoma* is found in the body's mucous membranes, while *ocular melanoma* usually begins as a small freckle in the eye.

The most common forms of melanoma are found on the leg, back, or face. They often develop from an existing mole, which can be triggered by excessive exposure to the sun. Early on, the melanoma doesn't form lumps or tumors. It isn't malignant, meaning it cannot yet spread to the internal organs and elsewhere. Yet, as we've seen, the melanoma lesion can spread down into the dermis layer; that's where it can begin to grow and metastasize throughout the body, lungs, brain, spleen, liver, heart, and, rarely, to the bone. The growth of the abnormal melanocytes can accelerate and spread, especially in older individuals.

Most moles are round, flat, and no larger than a pencil eraser. Few of these moles develop into melanoma. Still, about 20 percent of the white population can develop *dysplastic nevi* or atypical moles. (Fair-skinned individuals are often more prone to skin cancer because of the lack of melanin, which is a superb natural sunscreen.) Atypical moles differ markedly from common moles; they may be larger and can also be several shades of brown and even pink in color. They're also known for their irregular borders and inconsistent shape. These moles are the ones to keep an eye on, as changes in their appearance, in shape or color, make them candidates for removal and further examination by biopsy.

Babies are not usually born with moles, unless they have what are known as congenital nevi, a syndrome where large melanocytic lesions are present, sometimes covering the whole trunk. More "regular" moles will begin to appear in young children and teenagers. While most moles will never cause health problems, according to the American Cancer Society, someone with a great many moles is more likely to develop melanoma later in life.

So, if a dermatologist finds a spot or mole and suspects it could be cancerous—what comes next? The doctor may opt for a skin biopsy, which is done with a local anesthetic. Of course, this can be done for various forms of cancer. A bit of numbing medicine is injected into the area, and the doctor will either shave away the top layers of skin or use a cookie cutter–like tool to go slightly deeper into the skin. If the latter procedure is used, a few stitches may be necessary. In either case, only a small scar is the result.

If the tumor has grown deeper into the skin, the doctor will do an incisional biopsy, which removes a portion of the tumor, or perform an excisional biopsy, which removes the entire tumor, as well as a small outline of skin surrounding it.

When the melanoma is suspected to have spread further, nearby lymph nodes may be biopsied as well, to see whether any cancer has spread to them. Melanoma can spread quickly, perhaps reaching the lymph nodes, lungs, or brain while still being very small on the skin and at its original site. That's when CT scans and other imaging tests can better locate these more serious cancers.

A cancer's stage or staging helps doctors determine how serious the cancer is and decide how best to treat it. This is done by first determining the thickness of the tumor and how serious the ulceration, or breakdown of the skin, is over and around the melanoma.[14]

In Stage 0, the cancer is confined to the epidermis, the outermost layer of skin. In this case, it has not spread to any nearby lymph nodes or more distant parts of the body and can simply be removed without further treatments.

In Stage I, the tumor is no bigger than two millimeters, or

2/25ths of an inch. While it could be ulcerated, it's been determined that the cancer has not spread to the lymph nodes or elsewhere in the body.

In Stage II, the tumor is more than one millimeter in thickness, but it has not yet spread to distant parts of the body.

By Stage III, however, a number of classifications are added to each level. In this staging, the tumor is anywhere from one millimeter to four millimeters in thickness, but it may have spread to two or more nearby lymph nodes. In addition, it may have spread to small areas of nearby skin.

Stage IV is the highest and most dangerous level in melanoma and all cancers. Here, the major concern isn't necessarily the thickness of the tumor or whether it's ulcerated or even whether it's spread to nearby lymph nodes. The major characteristics of this high level is that the tumor has spread to *distant* lymph nodes and even on to such organs as the lungs, brain, and liver. The American Cancer Society reports that the five-year survival rate for many cancers has improved in recent years. Still, the survival rate for Stage IV melanoma is 25 percent.

SURVIVAL IS AT STAKE

As a tumor gets larger, it often outgrows its nutrient supply. When that happens, the tumor will send signals to blood vessels that are swimming by and say, "Hey, divert a branch over here," and then they'll grow new blood vessels into the tumor. That's a process we call angiogenesis.

Tumors can range from a few to thousands of cells. They can be cancerous (malignant) or noncancerous (benign). What's interesting is that the tumor, regardless of size, is clever enough to send them similar signals, ones that they would have during regular development. The endothelial cells, which cover the inner surface of the blood vessel, don't know any better and do what they're told, even if they're receiving signals from a tumor cell.

Cancer cells can move quickly when their survival is at stake. As we've seen, this is not a random process—this is what allows tumor cells to metastasize to distant sites. It can be a very aggressive situation. It's not as though they fall into the bloodstream and then settle somewhere else. Even when cancer cells move to a new location, their activity is much greater than what we knew about or realized a few years ago. When they do arrest in a new location, they move into the new tissue, including vital organs. And once they're there, they're intent on growing and surviving.

What we've learned in recent years is that not every organ is conducive to the outgrowth of every single type of cancer. There are different sites where cancer cells tend to go. For example, prostate cancer cells prefer to go to the bone; melanoma prefers to travel to the lung. Some of this movement is purely for physical reasons. A lot of cancer goes to the lungs or the liver because a lot of blood flows to those organs, carrying the tumor cells with it.

In other cases, it can depend upon what growth factors are being secreted. It's all about what the most conducive environments are for the tumor cells to grow. This has been coined the "seed and soil" hypothesis of cancer, where tumor cells (seeds) grow only in microenvironments conducive to them (soil). (Interestingly, this theory was proposed more than 130 years ago by Stephen Paget.)[15] To do this, they need to establish communication with the surrounding cells ("signaling") in their new environment, and it's those conversations that are so fascinating.

IMPORTANT CONVERSATIONS

How do cells talk to each other? This is a fascinating area of study that researchers are just beginning to understand. When people ask me, "Why haven't you cured cancer yet?" I reply, "Well, come spend a few days in the lab with me." That's where we're studying the ongoing conversations between cells. What we're overhearing and exploring can lead in many different directions. Through these "discussions," we're finding out more and more about cancer. In some ways, the work reminds me of the Sherlock Holmes and Famous Five mysteries I read as a kid. We're lab detectives.

Within the body, there are a great many conversations

going on daily, all at the same time. Cells in our fingertips signal to neurons in the brain that we just touched something hot or sharp, for example; cells exposed to the sun ask neighboring cells to protect them by making melanin. A tumor exists in a very complex neighborhood made up of a milieu of different cells, from immune cells, to fibroblasts ("the construction workers"), to blood cells. Fibroblasts may communicate directly through contact with each other, or indirectly, by releasing factors such as growth factors or fats, for example, or through little "bubbles" known as exosomes (more on that in a minute). Immune cells contribute to the conversation, not only by talking to the tumor cell, but by their complex interactions with each other as well. Often these immune cells are at odds with each other, the "bad" immune cells regulating and suppressing the "good" ones in a bid to allow the tumor to grow and colonize distant sites. One such example of the bad guys is the myeloid-derived suppressor cell. These cells can act not only to suppress immune activity in the tumor microenvironment, but also to forge new paths by going to distant sites where cells metastasize, to get the lay of the land, so to speak. The conversation may be something like, "All right, we're going to a lung to suppress the immune microenvironment there." That way the tumor cells can come in and not only survive but thrive. Other regulatory populations like T regulatory cells also have similar suppressive effects.

Fibroblasts are another critical part of the discussion.

THE LIFE CYCLE OF A CANCER CELL

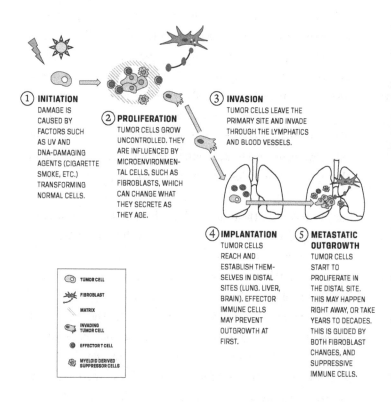

① INITIATION
DAMAGE IS CAUSED BY FACTORS SUCH AS UV AND DNA-DAMAGING AGENTS (CIGARETTE SMOKE, ETC.) TRANSFORMING NORMAL CELLS.

② PROLIFERATION
TUMOR CELLS GROW UNCONTROLLED. THEY ARE INFLUENCED BY MICROENVIRONMENTAL CELLS, SUCH AS FIBROBLASTS, WHICH CAN CHANGE WHAT THEY SECRETE AS THEY AGE.

③ INVASION
TUMOR CELLS LEAVE THE PRIMARY SITE AND INVADE THROUGH THE LYMPHATICS AND BLOOD VESSELS.

④ IMPLANTATION
TUMOR CELLS REACH AND ESTABLISH THEMSELVES IN DISTAL SITES (LUNG, LIVER, BRAIN). EFFECTOR IMMUNE CELLS MAY PREVENT OUTGROWTH AT FIRST.

⑤ METASTATIC OUTGROWTH
TUMOR CELLS START TO PROLIFERATE IN THE DISTAL SITE. THIS MAY HAPPEN RIGHT AWAY, OR TAKE YEARS TO DECADES. THIS IS GUIDED BY BOTH FIBROBLAST CHANGES, AND SUPPRESSIVE IMMUNE CELLS.

TUMOR CELL
FIBROBLAST
MATRIX
INVADING TUMOR CELL
EFFECTOR T CELL
MYELOID DERIVED SUPPRESSOR CELLS

These cells lay down the framework on which tumors grow, the cake stand if you will. They also act as teachers, instructing the behavior of the cancer cells, whether directly through secreted factors, or indirectly through microvesicles such as exosomes. Exosomes are like tiny bubbles full of lipids, proteins, and nucleic acids. They are released by all cell types and carry the hallmark of their cells of origin in their cargo, which can then travel throughout the body and be taken up by other cells. When fibroblasts and other cells release exosomes, that can dictate the behavior of the cancer cells that take them up. Whether the message is delivered directly, or packaged in an exosome, cells have ways of talking to each other, and these conversations dictate tumor cell behavior.

For example, we've recently shown in our research that older fibroblasts give fats to tumor cells, and the tumor cells receive that fat by expressing a transporter known as FATP2 on the surface of their cells.[16] Once they absorb that fat, they can use it to migrate and to resist therapy. Since our goal is to interrupt the conversations that drive tumors to be more aggressive, we interrupted this particular conversation by inhibiting the activity of FATP2 on tumor cells. When we did this, the cells, previously resistant to therapy, now became uniquely sensitive. Understanding how to harness, interrupt, or facilitate the conversations between the tumor and its environment, which changes as we age, is critical for effective cancer therapy. It takes us one step closer to learning how to make cancer deaths less inevitable after a diagnosis, or at least, we hope, to extending remission times.

CHAPTER 2

The Role
of Cancer Research

WHEN I WAS STUDYING CANCER in graduate school, I often thought, "Oh, my God, what are we dealing with here?" I learned how a cancer cell when treated with toxic drugs can build a "pump" on its surface to push the drugs back out. This multidrug resistance is now a well-known, well-characterized phenomenon. I watched the chromosomes inside cells break when given an over-the-counter chromium diet—broken chromosomes meant damaged DNA, and damaged DNA meant a tee-up for cancer. I watched melanoma cells morph into structures that look like blood vessels, a process called "vascular mimicry." Anyone who goes into cancer research has this epiphany, often multiple times over—where you're in awe, but you have a degree of trepidation, too, as you realize how cunning cancer is, and what measures must be taken against this opponent.

We've learned how adept cancer is at spreading throughout the body. Sometimes, the cancer is confined to a particular organ or area; in more cases the tumor will be detected in, say, the breast, but by the time a diagnosis is reached, the cancer will already have spread to other areas—the lungs, the bones, the brain. Even if we're able to determine whether the cancer is localized or has spread, it can be a fine line between what is too little and too much for a cancer patient to bear, especially in the pursuit of finding and ridding the body of every cancer cell.[1] If that isn't done, the cancer almost always returns and the patient suffers a relapse.

In the mid-1960s, a small group of doctors treating leukemia in children decided to test the limits in that area of cancer research. Sidney Farber, the father of chemotherapy, had great success at Children's Hospital in Boston treating kids with leukemia with a folic acid–blocking agent.[2] It was the first time a drug tested as an anticancer agent proved effective against leukemia. Despite such progress, Farber was reluctant to give children higher or potentially more dangerous doses. In addition, he resisted giving kids several chemotherapy drugs at the same time. "I will not injure two children to save one," he said. So it was left to other doctors in this field—Donald Pinkel, James Holland, Tom Frei, Emil Freireich, and others—to push the envelope when it came to chemotherapy. They began to prescribe such drugs increasingly in combination, what we call the chemotherapy "cocktail" today. "To really do the job, you need a combination of agents," Pinkel said. "Using them two, three, four at a time. That was a very fundamental observation and fundamental insight. It became key to our progress moving forward."[3]

For a few years in the 1960s, these cancer doctors were together at the Roswell Park Hospital in Buffalo, New York. Even when Pinkel left to establish St. Jude Children's Research Hospital in Memphis, the group still gathered several times a year. In part, that was because they were receiving so much criticism from their peers and the rest of the medical community about their new approach. "To many in the medical establishment, we were seen as reckless or even irresponsible," Jerry Yates said. "That resulted in many of the names that they called us—killers, poison pushers, renegades, pirates, cowboys. For a long time, we were shunned, ostracized by the rest of our world. That's how far out of bounds, even dangerous, we were perceived to be by others."[4]

Despite the harsh criticism, these "cowboys" continued conducting their clinical trials and publishing their reports, and eventually they took childhood leukemia from the 10 percent survival rate it had a half-century ago to the nearly 90 percent survival rate it has today. They are now recognized as cancer pioneers, and their success is a perfect, inspiring example of how research can lead to defying what seems to be a nearly inevitable, tragic outcome for thousands of families.[5]

PAYING MY DUES

Early in my career at Johns Hopkins, as a technician in the oncology center when I was barely 21 years old, it began to dawn on me that with cancer it isn't necessarily the initial tumor that kills you. Rather, it's how cancer can metastasize and spread throughout the body. I became fascinated with how cells move—what draws them to different sites. In addition, I realized that to do the kind of work that I wanted to do, I needed to go to graduate school.

Although as a woman during a less equitable era I'd received conflicting messages about far I could or should go in medicine, when I told Bob Casero, my boss at the Johns Hopkins Oncology Center, that I wanted to run my own lab someday, he couldn't have been more encouraging. Now I realize how unusual that was—perhaps still is. Bob confirmed that to go down this path, I'd need to attend graduate school, and he then helped me through the application process and wrote a recommendation. He urged me to talk to as many people as I could and learn about everything that was out there. He's been in my corner ever since.

Early on in that process, I was talking with another doctor—a gruff, old-fashioned guy, and he asked why I thought I needed a PhD. I told him how I was really interested in cancer research and how deeply I felt about the oncology patients with whom I'd worked. I told him how I had read books to the kids in the oncology ward at Johns Hopkins, and how much their plight touched me.

"Well, why don't you just become an MD?" he replied.

At first, I didn't know what to say. So I was honest and said, simply, "I don't have the emotional strength to do that on a daily basis. I need to bring about change for them from behind the bench." He looked at me and said, "That's one of the best answers I've ever heard." From then on, I knew to embrace my authenticity and be honest—be myself, for better or worse.

Around this time, Hopkins changed its rules for visa applications and procedures. I was in the United States on an F-1 student visa. I couldn't file for my green card as a technician—I had to be in a more senior position. By the time this happened, I'd missed all the application deadlines for doctoral programs at Hopkins and the vast majority of other schools. Then a strange thing happened.

I was going home one evening, feeling very discouraged about the visa and the graduate school situation, and when I got to my door found a flyer from George Washington University. I don't know whether someone, maybe a GW alum, slipped it under the door—there were a lot of students in my building, after all. However it got there, I was glad to get my hands on it. I couldn't believe it when I saw that they were offering rolling admissions and accepting students through June. They had a new PhD program in molecular and cellular oncology, which sounded tailor-made for me.

I applied and got an interview, which I'm pretty sure was because eminent scientists like Bob Casero and Bert Vogelstein wrote recommendations for me. In fact, when I went to Washington, DC, for the interviews, several of the professors there really only wanted to talk about Bert and the landmark work he was doing at the time! A little background is called for here. In the early 1990s, Bert and I once worked at the same location down on Bond Street at Hopkins. The building was an old grocery store that had been converted into labs. Bert was the first to unravel the genetic evolution of colon cancer. His identification of mutations of a gene known as p53 in colon cancer began a tide of research linking alterations in the gene and other cancers.[6] In 2003, he was ranked as the most highly cited scientist in the world during the previous 20 years.

During this time, I was also taking classes at the School of Public Health—in the department I now chair, ironically. One of the courses I had was in molecular carcinogenesis, and Bert was scheduled to be a guest lecturer in that course. I went to class that day, and the other students and I waited, and we waited, and we waited. But Bert never showed up. And I thought, "Wow, that's so uncool. Guess some people just think they're too big for their shoes." If you know Bert at all, you know how wrong I was about that! Remember this is the man who dedicated every textbook he ever wrote to his trainees, only accepts talks if trainees invite him, and so on. But back then, I didn't know him at all.

I was so mad that my sense of injustice got all fired up. I fumed all the way back to the lab. I had to go to a different room to develop the experiment I was working on, and when I walked in, there was Dr. Vogelstein, as I called him then.

"Oh, you're here?" I exclaimed.

"Excuse me?" he replied.

Now, you need to know this was the first time I'd ever talked to Bert Vogelstein. He didn't know me from a bar of soap.

I said, "Well, I just want you to know that there was a room full of students who were extremely disappointed you didn't show up. I've never seen students wait so long for a professor." Then I turned and left. (I'm a lot less impetuous these days.)

The next morning, I came into the lab, and as soon as I came through the door, someone said, "Bert Vogelstein has been here three times looking for you."

"Oh, God," I thought, "What have I done? I'm going to get fired." But I decided I might as well face the music, so I went across the hall to find him. He was just walking in to find me, and the first thing he did was ask my name. Then he said, "I just want you to know what happened. The invitation to your class had the wrong zip code. The envelope arrived the day of the lecture, and my assistant knew I wouldn't be able to do it, so she just put it away. I had no idea."

Bert went through this whole long explanation, and all the while I'm thinking, "Oh my God, you're Bert Vogelstein, why are you explaining yourself to me, a 20-year-old technician?"

But I kept my mouth shut. I let him go through the whole explanation.

At the end, I quipped, with a naughty smile, "OK, but don't let it happen again."

Bert cracked up, and so did I, and he's been my supporter and mentor ever since, guiding me through each transition of my entire career, to this very day. Many years later, when I got engaged to my husband, who had been a postdoctoral fellow in his laboratory, he quipped, "Well done, man; you've got a lively one there!" I think he was just too nice to say, "Good luck, you'll need it!"

So, I got accepted to George Washington University, and I began classes there late in the summer of 1994. From the beginning, I knew that I'd landed in the right place. I did my first rotation in the lab at GW, and I liked it so much that I told my advisor, who was also the head of the program, that I wasn't that interested in doing the usual rotations in multiple other laboratories. I just wanted to stay here, in the lab; he said, that's fine, and that's what I did.

Steve Patierno was my mentor at the university. We called him "Papa" Patierno because we were like his kids, and he always kept an eye out for us. It so happened that I was one of two people in his laboratory *not* working on chromium-induced molecular carcinogenesis, which is how cancer forms in the body upon exposure to chromium. As a result, I was able to focus on metastasis, which was where I wanted to be. From there I became particularly interested in the microenvironment because of how it guides metastasis. And to do that, I needed to understand how cells signal each other—the intracellular signaling we discussed in the previous chapter. The more I explored all of this, the more I became convinced that our bodies are hardwired somehow in this way and that the metastasis side of research was where to be.

After graduating from George Washington in 1998, I became a postdoctoral fellow at the Johns Hopkins Oncology Center. I had been working on prostate cancer since graduate school and was excited to postdoc at Hopkins with John Isaacs, a world leader in the field of prostate cancer. I thought that prostate cancer was going to be my specialty, where I'd make my mark. That's what I thought until Jeff Trent came into my life.

At the time, Jeff was the scientific director of the National Human Genome Research Institute at the National Institutes of Health in Bethesda, Maryland. He was a pioneer in the field of microarray design and pharmacogenomics, which is the study of how genes influence a person's response to drugs, and how drugs affect gene expression. This was all really new and exciting back then. After hearing his talk and seeing how kind he was to me in a meeting, I knew that I wanted to work with him and learn more about that field, too.

When I got to his lab, I told him, "I've been working on prostate cancer since grad school. I'd like to continue that." Jeff replied, "Well, the only problem is that I hired you because you're a cell biologist. And there's a new project I need your help on. If you want to come back to prostate cancer, it's fine. But for right now, I really need your help with this."

That project became our landmark study about Wnt5A in melanoma. Wnt5A is one of a family of proteins that can influence much of how the body reacts and deals with cancer.[7] The Wnt family, and specifically one member of that group of proteins, is key in allowing melanoma cells to resist therapy. It can also allow the cancer to leave the primary site and travel to metastatic sites elsewhere in the body.

It's funny. If Jeff hadn't said I could go back to prostate cancer at some point, who knows what would have happened. Would I have taken the job, this work that changed my life? I don't know, but I'm glad I did. Jeff taught me the value of collaboration, and working for him introduced me to melanoma research; that's where I've stayed ever since.

His lab had compared the gene expression patterns of melanomas that responded to early forms of immunotherapy to those that did not, using microarray technology.[8] Jeff wanted me to do a follow-up study to see how different gene expression patterns were potentially impacting metastasis, how all of this was affecting therapy resistance, different outcomes in patients, and how much of this hinged on the Wnt5A gene. It turned out to be a fascinating protein and a career-changing project. In many ways, we're still at work on these developments and insights today.

I joined the lab on October 2, 2000, just after I'd turned 30 and gotten engaged to my husband, Pat Morin. New job, new decade, new life. That's enough for now, right? But the world wasn't done with me quite yet. Three days after I took the job and began to commute from Baltimore to Bethesda, my dad passed away in Sri Lanka. (My parents had moved back there from Africa just that year.) As you know, I was really close to my dad. And it was very sudden. He was only 66 at the time. Unfortunately, he was a heavy smoker, and he had a triple abdominal aortic aneurysm. In the Western world, he might have survived that. But in Sri Lanka, 20 years ago, it was too quick, too much.

For someone like me to leave the country under those conditions isn't easy. To unexpectedly be called home can be complicated when you're an immigrant, because every time you leave the country, you need to have your visa papers in order. Since I had just started at Jeff's lab, much of my visa paperwork was up in the air. Thankfully, Pat took care of the details, while I crumbled under the news. We met my brother and sister in London and then flew together to Sri Lanka. When I returned to the United States, Jeff was there for me, too. I'd been working in his lab for only two days when my father died; then I'd been gone for nearly two weeks, with the time it took to get to Sri Lanka and back. So once we got back to Baltimore, I went straight to work the next day in Bethesda. Almost as soon as I came in, Jeff saw me and asked, "Why are you here?"

And I thought, "Oh God, he's firing me now. Because I disappeared for two weeks."

I jumped in with, "It's okay, I'll get to work. I'll work really hard."

And Jeff said, "No, I want you to go home. You've had a major life event. You need to process this, and you're not going to do it here."

We argued, with me insisting that I needed to stay—that work was the only way I could take my mind off what had happened. In the end, we made a deal. Jeff let me handle it my way, but he insisted that moving forward, the two of us would go out to lunch on a regular basis. He wanted to know what was on my mind, how I was working through this, how I was doing.

At first, I didn't think anything of it. I worked that day in the lab and was back again the next morning, eager to settle into some kind of routine. Yet a few weeks later, Jeff reminded me that we needed to catch up over lunch. He did this even though he was so busy at the time. I mean, he was the scientific director of the National Human Genome Research Institute! Right when they had just finished sequencing the human genome project! Every time you stepped off the elevator, there were reporters everywhere. We ran into Mike Wallace several times. It was just crazy.

Still, Jeff made the time, and whenever he took me to lunch, we didn't talk that much about the science. He wanted to hear about my dad. The work that he had done in Africa and elsewhere. I told him silly anecdotes, like how when I'd first started working at Hopkins as a young tech, my dad bragged about his daughter at Hopkins to everyone whom he met, even though I was basically just washing the dishes at the time!

Years later, when I was offered my current job at Johns

Hopkins, I called Jeff to ask what he thought. What was his advice? Was this the time for me to move? Was I ready for this level of a leadership job?

The first words out of Jeff's mouth were, "Oh, Ashi, Hopkins? All I can think is how proud your dad would have been." I couldn't believe he remembered my little anecdote how absurdly proud my dad was of my technician job at Hopkins, and it took me a few minutes to stop crying. I am so lucky—caring mentors like Steve, Bob, and Jeff have been the buttresses of any success I've had.

CANCER RESEARCH AS FOUR-DIMENSIONAL CHESS

As I said, I was planning to return to research in prostate cancer at some point. Yet in Jeff's lab, I became more intrigued by the work we were doing with the Wnt family of proteins. This is what eventually led me to the study of melanoma.

Compared with other areas of research in cancer, the field of melanoma was so embracing and inclusive. It didn't matter if you were a man or a woman, white or a person of color. My colleagues were a diverse, engaging group of international and domestic researchers. Everyone was so friendly and collaborative, an atmosphere created by the leadership at the time, specifically Meenhard Herlyn, who later became my close friend and colleague at The Wistar Institute. To this day, some of my closest friends and best collaborators are people I've met through this community.

The science was as stimulating as the community and the company. In my lab at the National Institute on Aging, we began to study a fascinating phenomenon in melanoma that runs counter to much of what we had understood about cancer up to this point. In a lot of cancers, if a tumor grows fast, it's also very aggressive. In melanoma, what we see is that tumors that have rapid growth tend to be less effective at leaving that primary site and metastasizing, going to other parts of the body. We call this the "Grow or Go" paradox, where a melanoma cell that otherwise has all of the indications of rapid growth tends to have fewer indicators of invasion, and vice versa. This isn't what we expected to find in our research several decades ago. That's what makes this family of proteins, the Wnts, so interesting in how they can influence cancer development. We started to realize that these proteins are absolutely critical—both in the early stage of the tumor as it begins to grow and develop, and in the later stages, when it leaves the primary site of the skin to invade the body. Through our studies of Wnt, we started to understand how different members of the same family of genes could play opposing roles, and yet both contribute to tumor progression.

In Jeff's lab, we had investigated Wnt5A, a member of that Wnt family. At that time, and even to this day to some extent, when you mention the term Wnt, most people's minds jump straight to the best-known mediator of Wnt signaling, a protein known as beta-catenin. Beta-catenin was made famous for its roles in colon cancer, in a paper out of Bert Vogelstein's lab that has been cited thousands of times.[9] The lead author of that paper, Pat J. Morin, was the man I would later marry, and he was the first to identify activating b-catenin mutations in cancer. But my work on Wnt signaling showed something different— not only did Wnt5A *not* activate beta-catenin in our melanoma systems; it actually suppressed it, through a different mechanism that did not involve its usual degradation pathway.[10]

Back then, this was uncharted territory for those of us in the field. Until this point, Wnt5A hadn't been associated with melanoma at all. Further studies from my laboratory have shown that this molecule is a key driver of metastasis. Wnt5A is critical in fostering changes in the cytoplasm's network of protein filaments and promoting different ways of invasion, ways we hadn't even considered nearly two decades ago. Others in the field are now also finding Wnt5A as a critical mediator of therapy resistance.

Our report was titled "Wnt5A signaling directly affects cell motility and invasion of metastatic melanoma." Although we'd presented the data publicly several times previously, the major presentation was scheduled for the American Association for Cancer Research meeting, which is held annually.

Until this point, the Wnt group had been seen as a signaling pathway for cancer, a family of proteins that drives cancer growth. And now here we were saying it didn't work that way with melanoma—Wnt5A didn't lead to a high proliferative/low invasive situation. In fact, it was the opposite: Wnt5A disables the beta-catenin pathway, slowing the cancer's growth but resulting in the cancer becoming invasive, much more prone to metastasis. Like anything that runs counter to prevailing opinions and beliefs, some people were intrigued by the new findings, while others got pretty upset about them.

Before our research, Wnt5A had largely been studied only in frogs. Randall Moon at the University of Washington outlined how it was a driver of the way frogs develop and the way that vertebrae line up and the embryos are formed.[11] It hadn't been fully studied in human beings, but that didn't stop some in my field from refusing to consider our data initially. Those people would say, "Wait a minute. It's a Wnt protein, so it must be driving growth." They insisted that if it's a Wnt, it should activate beta-catenin and be working through those pathways in the body. It was so new that not everyone could wrap their minds around it.

In looking back on it, we had a very naïve view of what these proteins can do, and the more we learn about Wnt5A, the more it surprises. At first, we thought that Wnt5A drove metastasis, end of story, but now we know that there is much more to it. Not just the expression of Wnt5A but where and when it is expressed are critical for tumor metastasis. For example, it's now known that tumor cells leave the primary site early and go to distant organs, like the lungs, and then just sit there for years, in this slow cycling state. Multiple changes can occur that then bring those cells out of that dormant state, and they start to grow. When that happens, they can soon become a problem, with large metastatic outgrowths to which patients eventually succumb. This emergence from dormancy can involve everything from secreted growth factors to changes in the immune system.

With melanoma, we've learned that this Wnt signaling pathway plays a huge role in driving such movement, via this "Grow or Go" paradox. Melanoma cells can switch between high proliferative / low invasive and low proliferative / high invasive phenotypes, which is guided by changes in Wnt signaling. So, cells need to stop growing and start going to leave the primary site, but when they get to the distant organ, they need to pause and make sure they can survive that new environment.[12]

In the lab, we began to see that a cancer cell that's multiplying rapidly, driven by beta-catenin, has a lot of antigens, the substances that cause the immune system to produce antibodies against what it has determined to be an intruder or invader. Antigens can get presented as red flags to the immune system on the surface of the cell. In other words, the immune system doesn't recognize the cell's products and sees them as foreign. In essence, they're signaling to the immune cells to come in and attack. But we found that Wnt5A can shut much of that down.

In doing so, Wnt5A can hide the tumor from the immune system very effectively. It's part of how it helps the cell survive its new environment. Our most recent work is leading us to realize, though, that changes in that new environment eventually conspire to suppress that Wnt5A-driven dormant phenotype, and drive reactivation of the "grow" program, such that those cells start to grow out again, forming large metastatic outgrowths.

Someone once said that cancer research can be like playing three-dimensional chess. But our work, and that of others reveals that it's at least four-dimensional chess—with time being a critical piece of the puzzle. I will always be grateful to Jeff for letting me take the Wnt5A story and pursue it as my own research. Had he not left the National Human Genome Research Institute to move to Arizona, I would have loved to continue pursuing that work with him. But that was not to be, and when he moved to Arizona, I accepted an offer from the National Institute on Aging.

MOVING ON TO THE NATIONAL INSTITUTE ON AGING

In 2004, I became a staff scientist at the National Institute on Aging (NIA) in Baltimore. Even though I struggled with some of the personalities there and the machinations required just to get my job done (many a night I drove home after work in tears), during my eight years at NIA I began to explore the important role that aging plays in cancer. While I didn't actually work on aging during my time at NIA, this is where my interest in aging's influence on cancer, specifically melanoma, took off, thanks in part to conversations with Dan Longo, our brilliant scientific director at the time.

Working at the NIA was challenging. I wasn't on tenure-track, and to earn my keep if you will, I helped to manage a large laboratory that focused on research that was beyond my area of expertise. What kept me going there was my own tiny group of three or four people. We did the research I was interested in, and I was able to write senior author papers and have them published. Our work was becoming more recognized, especially in the international melanoma community. I had once thought that cancer research would always be kind of competitive, which at times turned me off. Yet the international melanoma community continued to win me over with their offers of support and collaboration. I was now, and have remained ever since, Team Melanoma, my prostate cancer study days long forgotten.

Despite the challenges at NIA, there were so many positives, from wonderful colleagues to being exposed to people like Judith Campisi and her work on senescence. A senescent cell is one that basically stops growing but doesn't die. It may seem like these kinds of cells are just sitting there, but they're in fact secreting several different factors that are crucial to cancer development. Judy identified that what these cells are secreting can be a double-edged sword. Some of them are immunological factors and can be tumor suppressive. But others act as signals to the cell to metastasize and/or grow.[13]

Over the years, we found that there are very different types of senescence. One of the types that my lab identified a few years ago was called "pseudo senescence." That's when the cells look like they're senescent—aging, becoming more inactive—but they can be very invasive. They can metastasize to different sites, and as we age these processes become more pronounced.

That aging would have a major influence upon cancer seems a bit obvious today, but we never really thought too deeply about it until a few years ago. The microenvironment—what's happening around the tumor and how it affects the tumor—has become a major part of my thinking and research philosophy. So much so that I believe that it also applies to the world and people right around you, around each of us—your actions, your decisions, the way you respond to things. In many ways, our very behavior with regard to our immediate surroundings can function like cells in our body.

While I'd never thought about aging and cancer that much until I took the job at NIA, once there, with everybody around me working and thinking about aging, I thought, "Wait a minute, maybe all of these aging changes that are occurring normally drive the aggression of cancer as a disease of aging? Let me look at that more closely."

So, even though it was difficult at times personally, my years there were a huge leap forward for me and my research about cancer. Now we realize that older people get cancer in large part because they often have deteriorating immune systems, that they're at a great risk of developing genetic mutations over time—that aging was a major prognostic factor for cancer. My time at NIA sowed the seeds of my work on aging and cancer, and then I joined The Wistar Institute, where that work flourished.

CHAPTER 3
Breaking Through

IN 2011, AFTER EIGHT YEARS at the National Institute on Aging, I was ready to make a major move, and my daughter, Alina, was old enough that I could now do this, even though I knew she would struggle with missing our neighborhood and her friends. I knew I was asking a lot of my husband, too. After leaving Hopkins, Pat had started his own lab at the National Institutes of Health focusing on ovarian cancer. He was the first to discover that proteins called claudins, which normally acted as tight junctions between cells, were altered in ovarian cancer, allowing the cancer cells to pick up and metastasize.[1] Abnormal claudin expression was then found in breast cancer and is now a factor that is considered in the staging of breast cancers.

Although Pat's work was flourishing, he sensed that I needed to be around more researchers who were specifically studying melanoma and other skin cancers, so he encouraged me to accept a new position as an assistant professor in the molecular and cellular oncogenesis program at The Wistar Institute in Philadelphia, an independent nonprofit research institution on the campus of the University of Pennsylvania focusing on the biomedical sciences. For nearly two years I commuted between Baltimore and Philadelphia, and eventually we made the move north.

Wistar was a new and empowering beginning for me. For the first time, I was allowed to do my research independently, with my own resources to allocate as I saw fit. It was so different from being at NIA because I was in charge of the direction of my laboratory, and as long as I got the grant funding to do so, I could study whatever I wanted. It was my first experience with grant writing, and I absolutely loved it. Each grant serves as a blueprint for the next few years of scientific direction. Then and now, I love thinking through the problems I want to solve, coming up with experiments and plans on how to do so, and then receiving both criticism and positive feedback from colleagues on what would work, what would most certainly fail, and how it all needs to be communicated. My colleagues didn't hold back—if they didn't agree with the data presented, they would say so. But in the next breath, they'd say, "If you really want to answer that question, you need to use these models. I have many, and I'd be happy to share them with you." Their disagreement wasn't rooted in criticism, but in their commitment to having everything studied as accurately as possible. You received the brutally honest critiques— and sometimes those stung—but you also got the support you needed to move ahead. That's what made Wistar a crucial place in my development as a cancer researcher. The specific expertise of my colleagues, the research freedom, the abundant feedback, and the heavy emphasis on grant writing there all made Wistar a turning point in my research.

Within three years, I was named an associate professor in tumor microenvironment and metastasis, and I eventually became the program co-leader in immunology, microenvironment, and metastasis. By adding aging to the overall picture, we were making strides in our ability to one day manage and control more facets of cancer—to work against some of its current inevitabilities. I knew we were on the verge of major discoveries, and I felt like I was opening a treasure chest and pulling out one insight after another. We soon realized that several of the processes of cancer and aging, which appeared to be in opposition sometimes or have little in common other times, were actually shared by the disease. Such hallmarks include cellular survival, metabolic changes, decreased fitness, and an abnormally high rate of proliferation of rapidly dividing cells. We also began to see how intracellular communications, mitochondrial dysfunction, cellular senescence, and other key factors could be shared by the majority of cancers. We observed that normal cells "talked" to cancer cells and that cancer cells responded, but also, critically, that the types of conversations the cells had changed with age.

Sometimes in research, a seemingly simple shift you make away from a tried-and-true, decades-old practice can make a

The Business Side of Research

It's always thrilling to learn about major scientific and technological breakthroughs in the news—of the promise of new treatments and even cures, exciting new discoveries, and inventions that solve long-standing problems and make our lives easier. But even for researchers at leading research institutions like Johns Hopkins University, with our state-of-the-art labs and field stations and highly trained, inspiring colleagues, there are obstacles that make those victories more difficult, including securing immigrant scientists' visas (discussed on page 60), the cost of funding laboratory personnel, and the complexities and high fees associated with publishing findings of the research.

As with most businesses, operating income is a primary concern for laboratory work. Most researchers are reliant upon grants from the government and philanthropic foundations to complete their studies, which requires equipment, materials, staffing, and more. But some of the major sources of financial support, including the National Institutes of Health, haven't increased their funding amounts for individual grants in the last thirty years, and annual modular budgets remain at $250,000 per grant. During this same period, salaries for graduate students and postdoctoral fellows have doubled—which is welcome news. But to pay them, lab directors have to spend much more time writing and applying for ever more grants to supplement their finances, which is an enormously time-consuming (and nerve-wracking) job—even though thinking through what the proposed project's experiments could reveal, and what work is necessary to get to those revelations, can be an exciting, creative process.

Another major consideration of research is the increasingly high bar set for publications, and the associated costs. If you think back to the 1953 *Nature* paper by James Watson and Francis Crick describing the structure of DNA, it was exactly one page long, with one figure composed of a single panel. Today, articles for that journal involve so much more. Our 2016 *Nature* paper (discussed on page 51), for example, included a total of fourteen figures (five main, nine supplementary), each with multiple panels of data. Further, the publishing costs alone—in addition to the research costs—of a single article in such leading journals can run a lab as much as $10,000. This is particularly true if you want the piece to be open access—to share it with as wide an audience as possible—which puts smaller labs doing great work on limited budgets at a disadvantage in getting their work recognized and accessed widely.

On the bright side, this has driven a positive change in recent years toward collaborative grant writing, where multiple labs nationwide and even worldwide apply for grants together, bettering their odds for successful applications. I'm a big believer that diversity at every level, from gender to race to ways of thinking, is critical in finding creative solutions to solve and better understand cancer, so bringing in other teams is a great way to overcome some of the roadblocks while gaining the best understanding of the problems at hand.

big difference. One of the basic changes we made in our lab as we started at Wistar in 2011 was the age of the mice we were working with. The mice we were using at first were six to eight weeks old, which is the age that most researchers work with. But when you equate that to humans, that's only 14 to 16 years old, and it makes little sense if you're trying to study how cancer works in patients ages 65 and older.[2] So, in my lab, we used mice for our research that were 12 months to 18 months old, which correlate much better to older human beings. That's the human equivalent of 50 to 70 years old.

Soon after we made this switch, we noticed that if we treated younger mice and older mice with many of the same cancer drugs, the two groups responded much differently. At first, we focused on tumors and specific genetic mutations. For example, we had a drug that targeted a particular genetic mutation, and we put those tumors in young mice. Then we put the same tumors in the older mice, and we gave both the same drug. The tumors in the young mice soon went away, but the tumors in the older mice grew during the treatment. It was becoming more apparent to us that targeting age-related changes in cancer would provide novel and intriguing new paths of therapy and care.

When it came to aging, and the role it plays in cancer, I was lucky to be in the right place at the right time. I now had a foot in cancer research at Wistar, and after my work at the National Institute on Aging, I had my other foot in aging research. It was natural for me to explore the intersection of these two worlds. As I did so, I realized that while I'd been surrounded by researchers focused on aging during my eight years at NIA, they weren't really thinking about cancer, or its microenvironment, which was becoming a much bigger part of my thinking. Certainly, genetic changes are important. But so is the microenvironment that informs and impacts the cancer.

Mina Bissell is one of my heroes who's done amazing work in this area. Born in Tehran, Iran, she's another feisty immigrant who's made her mark in the medical world. She's the former head of life sciences at the Lawrence Berkeley Laboratory in California, and in researching breast cancer she's made major breakthroughs in our understanding of the microenvironment and tissue architecture. I first heard Mina speak when I was 20 years old, at the American Association for Cancer Research meeting in Washington, DC. It's an annual meeting, attended by a large number of cancer researchers from all over the world—about 20,000 of us. She discussed the microenvironment and how you could take a prostate cell and turn it into a milk-producing mammary cell, simply by changing the environment in which it was set. It was fascinating because it demonstrated how such cell plasticity could be another major factor in our understanding of cancer biology and how to better eliminate tumors.

In a popular TED Talk she gave in 2012, Mina emphasized how puzzling deciphering cancer's form and function can be given that we have upward of 70 trillion cells in our body.[3] Mina's research revealed that the microenvironment and extracellular matrix can tell the cancer cells what to do. In essence, the cancer's growth and malignant behavior is regulated at the level of tissue organization, and tissue organization is dependent on the extracellular matrix and microenvironment.

Mina uses the term "dynamic reciprocity" to describe the conversations cells are having with each other—how the normal cells are sending chemical signals—communicating to the tumor cells—and the tumor cells are talking back to the normal cells. It's similar in many ways to the back and forth in conversations we participate in during everyday life. Mina's work was groundbreaking in its challenge of existing paradigms, and it inspired my own work on the tumor microenvironment in trying to interpret these conversations.

At Wistar, the developments and insights we were gaining regarding correlations between cancer and aging were complex and challenging to fully comprehend, but we were increasingly enthusiastic about what we were seeing. It took us seven years to put together the first set of data because we wanted to be absolutely sure of everything. We were seeing the major influences aging has, especially once we switched to older mice, and some of these changes could be queried in patient samples—for instance, the expression of proteins that changed in aging human skin as well as mouse skin, or similar responses (or lack thereof) to therapy in both older mice and older humans. As we continued, it became absolutely clear that aging is an important characteristic of cancer, especially in older patients.

"Cancer is a disease of aging." That was the opening line in a landmark study from my Wistar laboratory, published by *Nature* in 2016. While there are of course childhood cancers, they occur less frequently and are in general more curable. And while cancers that are more prevalent in older patients also strike younger patients, when we look at the disease as a whole, more than 70 percent of all cancers diagnosed worldwide are seen in individuals over the age of 65, and almost 90 percent of the deaths from cancer occur in the same age group.[4]

Our work in this initial study laid out techniques for focusing on molecular changes that occur in aging skin cells and understanding how those changes can drive melanoma metastasis and therapy resistance in older patients. Such insights shifted our views on how we should be treating patients with melanoma. In many ways, this initial study was the foundation of much that has followed with my research. The study wasn't completed that long ago, but when I look back on what we had just started to uncover, it amazes me how much we've learned so quickly: the impact of age on a few factors that play a role in tumor progression; the involvement of the aging immune microenvironment; how different organs age differently, which governs metastatic outgrowth; and the involvement of fats as well as proteins. The gratifying part has been identifying actionable changes, molecules we can target, to overcome some of this age-related therapy resistance, and we're anxious to introduce drugs that target these changes into the clinic.

In hindsight, the correlation between aging and cancer makes a lot of sense, given that cancer is basically defined as cell growth without normal barriers. We've learned that as we age, we accumulate more mutated, distorted genes that have been lying in wait. These can crowd out the normal genes, which perform vital cellular functions. Until only a few generations ago, many of us didn't live long enough for cancer to be a major problem. Diseases like cholera, smallpox, and tuberculosis were considered more dire because they usually impacted younger patients.

We often see major changes in how cancer can grow and move throughout the body in people 65 and older. While this was recognized, in part, by the National Cancer Institute and others a half-century ago, there were cost and complexity barriers to running trials and extensive investigations that extend over years and decades. Such longitudinal studies can be difficult to carry out and are sometimes prone to error as they take place over a longer period of time. That's why until recently there's been limited data from clinical trials in older patients. Only 40 percent of patients enrolled in cancer clinical trials were over 65, and fewer than 10 percent were over 75. As a result, age was often overlooked as a major factor in detecting and treating cancers like melanoma. Now we know it's as important as skin type, family history, and spending too much time in the sun.

What was common knowledge was that you're more prone to chronic inflammation as you grow older, which makes many people more vulnerable to a variety of different diseases as they age. But few researchers looked in-depth at what was going on at the molecular level—at how aging could alter and influence not only the tumor cells, but the surrounding cells as well. The incidence of cancer could escalate further as life expectancy continues to rise. That's the door we've begun to open, and what we're discovering gives hope to future therapy and care for many forms of cancer.

In that 2016 study, we focused on the role aging can specifically play in the development of melanoma. For example, melanoma patients 65 and older often have significantly higher serum levels of a protein known as sFRP2 than patients younger than 40. Secreted frizzled-related protein 2 is a protein that is encoded by the sFRP2 gene and an important factor with Wnt signaling. Elevated levels of sFRP2 can cause a decrease in beta-catenin and, ultimately, the loss of a key redox effector, or multifunctional protein, called APE1. The loss of APE1 can result in melanoma cells being more prone to DNA damage, more genetically unstable, and more resistant to therapy. Our findings in this study also supported the hypothesis that dynamic changes with an aged microenvironment play a key role in increasing resistance to therapy. With melanoma, mutations in the BRAF gene, a key driver of melanoma, are present in nearly 70 percent of patients under the age of 45. However, these tumors are less aggressive in younger patients and more responsive to targeted therapy. In the 2016 study we compared outcomes in patients who had been treated with the drug vemurafenib, which targets the BRAF mutation in melanoma. We obtained these data from multiple centers that had treated these patients, in the United States and other centers across the world. This study involved so many different centers that the final author count on the ensuing publication was more than 50! The most surprising thing to us was that at the start of this study, we didn't expect to find huge differences with age, because we were targeting a specific mutation (in the BRAF gene) with a drug designed to hit that mutant gene product. In our minds, nothing else should have mattered: one gene, one mutation, one drug. But instead, all of the changes that occurred with age combined to provide avenues for cells to escape that therapy and rendered it less effective in older patients. The study concluded, "Our data suggested that, as the general population ages, new efforts must be made to understand and treat cancer in an age-appropriate manner." That may seem like a simple statement, but this was a wholly new direction in cancer research.

Many of the key factors and processes were now established. The next step was to carry out the rigorous work to ensure that future data and insights were solid and indisputable—to build on this new knowledge in the smartest, most effective way.

Fibroblasts are the cells that are responsible for maintaining the extracellular matrix and for supporting cellular and microenvironmental homeostasis (the healthy state that is maintained by the constant adjustment of biochemical and physiological pathways). This is accomplished through the regulated secretions of cytokines, chemokines, growth factors and other key signaling proteins. Because we were studying a tumor in the skin, it made perfect sense to look at the fibroblasts as the orchestrator of those changes. Most of our studies focused on the interaction between fibroblasts and the melanoma cells. We soon realized that the age of the fibroblasts was critical in the impact they had on tumor cells. Previously, work from Judy Campisi's lab at the Buck Institute in California had shown that irradiating embryonic fibroblasts and making them senescent (mimicking aging) drove tumor progression.[5] To our knowledge, we were the first to isolate normal fibroblasts from younger versus older patients and assess their impact on melanoma cells. What our work found was that with age, these factors changed dramatically. Further, our work also showed that tumor cells didn't need to be in direct contact with fibroblasts in order to be influenced by them—we found that fibroblast-secreted factors were even more potent influencers of tumor behavior. That was important because it meant that these age-related changes could be systemic, impacting not only the primary tumor, but also metastases at different sites; this also meant that targeting these age-related changes could impact metastatic disease.

We've also learned that persistent inflammation can lead to tissue degeneration and is heavily associated with cancer induction and progression. One of the hallmarks of aging is an increase in systemic low-grade chronic inflammation, which occurs due to age-related changes in microbiota of the gut, genetics, chronic infections, cellular senescence, and other changes, termed "inflammaging." Cellular senescence is recognized as a key contributor in linking inflammaging with age-related malignancies. As Campisi detailed in a 2007 report, cellular senescence is a multifaceted process that arrests cell growth, and it can affect key tumor pathways controlled by p53 and retinoblastoma proteins.[6] Another element linked to inflammaging is the recruitment of a specific type of immune cell known as myeloid-derived suppressor cells (MDSCs). These cells can be potent repressors of effector T cells, which play a central role in our immune system, and MDSCs are associated with increased disease progression in cancer. We've studied how these and other subpopulations of immune cells (including T cells, natural killer cells, macrophages, and dendritic cells) change during the aging process. In older patients, cells such as neutrophils and macrophages appear to switch toward more immunosuppressive states. This can promote tumorigenesis, or the production of tumors, and is leading to an increased understanding of how the age-related changes in additional cells, immune cells, in the microenvironment contribute to tumorigenesis.

However, it's not a simple concept. For example, our immune system weakens as we grow older. Immunotherapy is the treatment of disease by activating or suppressing the immune system, and that's one of the main tools we use to fight cancers these days. But when you're dealing with immunotherapy, specifically immunotherapy that targets the checkpoints or regulators of the immune system, it turns out that a slightly weaker immune system can sometimes actually help, because the regulatory systems that would normally tamp down the immune response boosted by immunotherapy don't function as well. If you'd told me before we did these studies with older mice that they would respond better to this example of immunotherapy, I would have laughed. But they did. In these cases, having a weaker immune system is an unexpected advantage, which, of course, isn't usually the case with cancer. We showed that this was true in patients, where we studied approximately five hundred patient outcomes, and found that largely, older melanoma patients had better results than younger patients after treatment with immunotherapy.[7] These results have been validated by other researchers now, in much larger melanoma patient data sets, and with multiple forms of immunotherapy.[8] However, in other tumor types like breast cancer, work from Sandra McAllister's laboratory at Brigham & Women's Hospital finds this is not always the case, and older breast cancer patients do not respond as well to immunotherapy.[9] This dichotomy between tumor types further highlights the complexity of the impact of aging on cancer.

We continued to study and extrapolate the data, shifting the focus from mice to what happens in humans. It's been demonstrated that older patients' metastases can be further away from their cancer's origin site. In melanoma, we see that young patients develop more lymph node metastases than older patients, but older patients develop more of the deadly distal metastases (liver, lung, heart, brain) than younger patients. Our work has shown that in part, these different routes of metastasis occur because of changes in the aging microenvironment, many of which are orchestrated by the fibroblasts. Some of these changes are mechanical, meaning that the tumor cells in the older patients have more "room" to sneak into blood vessels, while other changes may be more molecularly driven, through changes in some of the growth or immune factors.

What we've learned in a few short years is that aging can amplify many factors governing cancer. The mechanisms between the disease and aging underscore the time-dependent aspect of cellular damage. Fibroblasts and immune cells appear particularly susceptible to this age-related impact. The data strongly indicate that we need a paradigm shift in our approach to aging and how it influences our understanding of cancer.

We'll need all of the best cancer research minds available to solve these puzzles—to determine better diagnostic methods and treatments to reduce even more of cancer's mortality rates.

THE PRICELESS ROLE OF IMMIGRANTS

I've been so fortunate to work with many incredible trainees. They're the engine that drives the research in the lab, and mentoring them is my greatest pride and joy. This is not to ignore the contributions of either the amazing immigrants who've gone before them, or the incredible American students who have spearheaded innovative research in my lab, and now in their own, such as Marie Webster, who was instrumental, along with fellow Americans such as Curt Kugel III, and other immigrant scientists like Aman Kaur and Michael O'Connell, in establishing my lab at Wistar. Before them came trainees from all over the world: Tura Camilli from France, Reeti Behera from India, even one trainee, Samudra Dissanayake from Sri Lanka where I was born, and another, Poloko Leotlela, from Lesotho where I grew up, and so many more! Currently in my lab I have two Black women scientists, two Latina scientists, and half of us are immigrant scientists. I have always been amazed at the deep friendships we form despite our cultural differences.

What is worrisome is that many of my international trainees first came to this country as I did on an F-1 or a J-1 scholarly visa. In recent years, such visa holders have been subjected to draconian restrictions, with paltry explanations provided for such treatment. These complications have occurred even though such visa holders are required to return to their own countries after five years here in the United States. Usually, they have to wait two years before being able to return.

Why do we need immigrant scientists in the United States? Why don't we simply rely on American-born professionals to fit the bill? The fact is, we don't have enough specialists to go around. Many labs in this country are looking for grad students, technicians, and postdoctoral fellows. By not fully filling those positions, we're limiting the science we can do right now. We're restricting what our labs and programs can accomplish here, in America, not just for medical research, but for the wider range of studies that move society forward. Hopefully, that will change with the recent shift in administrations in Washington.

I'm a firm believer that if you look at the same problem from every available angle, you're much more likely to find more innovative and creative solutions. Research demands a diversity of influences and streams of thought; one single approach, no matter how brilliant, will not defeat our deadliest and most debilitating threats, including cancer. Cancer cells are always changing, so we need to consistently hear from people with varied perspectives, experiences, educations, philosophies, and mindsets. Sometimes it takes a person from a different culture—perhaps one that's more communal or collective, where the communities are more dependent upon each other—to show us the way forward. When you look at the list of Nobel laureates in science and medicine since 1947, 43 percent of the American awardees were immigrants to this country (to read more, see page 63). They've demonstrably influenced the US labs they were a part of by changing the perceptions and outlooks of their coworkers, in addition to contributing pivotal scientific bodies of work.

Too few realize that immigrants have been such a major factor in US research through the years They may have read that Albert Bourla, the CEO of Pfizer, is a Greek immigrant, and that the CEO of Moderna, Noubar Afeyan, was born in Lebanon. One of the key scientists behind mRNA vaccines is Katalin Kariko, a Hungarian scientist. These and other immigrants have worked tirelessly to help save our nation from COVID-19, its worst health crisis in a century. But the collective impact of these immigrants across the research and health care fields is rarely discussed.

These scientists have helped to form the foundation of contemporary research; their work has saved, and will save, countless lives.[10] They also educate the next generation of scientists, further deepening their impacts. For instance, Carl and Gerty Cori were both born in Prague and came to the Roswell Park Cancer Institute in Buffalo in 1922, where they began groundbreaking work on tumor metabolism. In time, they moved to Washington University and built a department of biochemistry there, which included seven future Nobel laureates. Zena Werb was born in the Bergen-Belsen concentration camp in Germany in 1945. After World War II, her family

Immigrant Soldiers in the Battle

If we're going to manage, control, and even perhaps cure cancer one day, it will need to be a collaborative effort with all the most original, best-trained minds from around the world contributing their ideas and findings. But many scientists are alarmed about the restrictions fellow researchers and others in our fields have faced in recent years in trying to secure visas to the United States, and also in being forced to return to their home nations even though their work was not complete. They want to join us in this multifaceted campaign against cancer, to contribute to solutions, but face often insurmountable obstacles.

That's what inspired my husband, Pat Morin, Denis Wirtz, and me—all immigrants to America—to co-write a commentary on the subject in 2020 for *Cancer Cell* titled "Completing the Great Unfinished Symphony of Cancer Together: The Importance of Immigrants in Cancer Research." Pat is executive director of strategy and implementation at the Abramson Cancer Center in Philadelphia; Denis is vice provost for research and the Theophilus Halley Smoot Professor of Engineering Science at Johns Hopkins. Beyond our personal experiences, we all share a common respect for the contributions of our international students, colleagues, and staff members.

Few realize the enormous impact immigrants have had on US research through the years, beyond famous physicists including Enrico Fermi, Hans Bethe, and Albert Einstein, who came to this country and helped America win weapons and space races. Yet the pivotal immigrant factor goes far deeper in the sciences, and many other disciplines; cancer research is a perfect example. This list of 23 US Nobel laureates whose award-winning work contributed to cancer research illustrates a small percentage of the debt we owe to those who've been welcomed through our doors.

US IMMIGRANT NOBEL LAUREATES IN BIOMEDICAL RESEARCH, 1947–2015

Name	Nation of Origin	Year Awarded	Research Focus
Sidney Altman	Canada	1989	Catalytic properties of RNA
Baruj Benacerraf	Venezuela	1980	Genetic basis of immunology
Elizabeth Blackburn	Australia	2009	Telomerase co-discovery
Günter Blobel	Poland	1999	Protein transport
Mario Capecchi	Italy	2007	Gene targeting
Albert Claude	Belgium	1974	Electron microscopy
Gerty and Carl Cori	Austro-Hungary	1947	Cell metabolism
Max Delbrück	Germany	1969	DNA replication
Renato Dulbecco	Italy	1975	Cancer viruses
Charles Brenton Higgins	Canada	1966	Hormones in cancer therapy
Har Gobind Khorana	India	1968	Deciphering genetic code
Rita Levi-Montalcini	Italy	1986	Nerve growth factor
Fritz Lipmann	Germany	1953	Bioenergetics
Salvador Luria	Italy	1969	Genetic structure of viruses
Paul Nurse	England	2001	Cell cycle
Severo Ochoa	Spain	1959	RNA polymerase
George Emil Palade	Romania	1974	Electron microscopy
Aziz Sancar	Turkey	2015	DNA damage
Oliver Smithies	England	2007	Gene targeting
Ralph Steinman	Canada	2011	Dendritic cells
Jack Szostak	England	2009	Enzyme telomerase
Susumu Tonegawa	Japan	1987	Antibody production

After Morin, Wirtz, and Weeraratna 2020

emigrated to Canada, where she began college at the age of 16 and eventually moved to the University of California, San Francisco, where she initiated classic studies on the tumor environment, focusing on the extracellular matrix and tumor microenvironment. Other outstanding immigrant researchers in the field of tumor microenvironment include Mina Bissell (Iran), Kornelia Polyak (Hungary), Rakesh Jain (India), Mikala Engeblad (Denmark), Yibin Kang (China), and many others. Min Chiu Li emigrated from China to the University of Southern California in 1947 to pursue postgraduate education. He soon became part of the team at the National Cancer Institute developing modern chemotherapy.

The list of immigrant contributions goes on and on, and it involves all types of cancer research. The best and the brightest want to be here, in this country, because the top labs and top people are here. Many have brought new treatments to our shores, including Waun Ki Hong (from South Korea), Carlos Arteaga (Ecuador), Olufunmilayo Olopade (Nigeria), Gabriel Hortobagyi (Hungary), Irene Ghobrial (Egypt), Chi Van Dang (Vietnam), Jean-Pierre Issa (Lebanon), Lieping Chen (China), Baruj Benacerraf (Venezuela), Azra Raza (Pakistan), and Kristiina Vuori (Finland).

The contributions of these and other immigrant scientists helped form the foundation of my work at Wistar—and that of other cancer researchers around the globe—and continue to aid my work today. Our breakthroughs rest on their achievements.

CHAPTER 4

A Vision for Future Care

FRANKLY, I THOUGHT I'D BE AT WISTAR for decades. But in late 2018, Denis Wirtz, the vice provost for research and Theophilus Halley Smoot Professor of Engineering Science at Johns Hopkins University, reached out to me. Naturally I went to Baltimore and spoke with him, given the university's stature in medical research and my history there, but I was still thinking that I'd stay at Wistar. Denis is an expert in the molecular and biophysical mechanisms of cell motility and adhesion and nuclear dynamics in health and disease, and he's a high-energy, very positive person. He really wanted me to return to Hopkins, and I appreciated his interest and enthusiasm, but I told him that the timing wasn't right. Deep down, I wondered whether I was ready for that big a move. Perhaps my imposter syndrome was flaring up, especially since I had also been asked to consider not only the Bloomberg Professorship that Denis was offering, but also the Chair of Biochemistry and Molecular Biology at the School of Public Health. After my first recruitment visit, as impressed as I was by the department, the dean, and everyone

I'd met, I thought that I had more that I needed to do at Wistar, including seeing through a large multicenter translational grant I'd just submitted with the University of Pennsylvania. When I told Denis that I was going to stay at Wistar, he asked me not to do anything for a day or so, not to send anything out about this on email. Within hours, I'd heard from Ron Daniels, the president of the university, and scheduled a visit with Paul Rothman, dean of Medicine, and a second visit with Ellen MacKenzie, the dean of the Bloomberg School of Public Health. The persuasion committee was at work, which became hard to resist.

Ellen set up a second round of talks in Baltimore, and this time I spoke with Baltimore's former deputy health commissioner, Josh Sharfstein, about melanoma awareness programs. Throughout my career, I've spoken with schoolchildren about the need for sun protection and the dangers of tanning beds. During my time at Wistar, I initiated a chain of events that resulted in the distribution of sunblock dispensers in the Philadelphia area. Ellen had done her homework, and she knew how important local efforts are to me—that it's necessary that we take the insights we're discovering in the lab and bring them to the general public in a timely manner. I also spoke with Nobel Prize laureates and other department chairs who lived in Philadelphia and commuted to Baltimore. Instinctively, Ellen knew that some of my reservations were about how this would affect my family, and she so beautifully planned that second visit around all of my interests and concerns.

Another important conversation I had the second time around was with Paul Rothman, the dean of the medical faculty. "I'm not saying we're going to do it or even can do it," he told me. "But let's say you had unlimited resources. What would you do with them? What's your vision?" Of course, this is one of those open-ended questions that can come up in such situations. But I already knew that what I really wanted to do one day is to build the world's first true cancer and aging center, which is what I told him. "An aging and cancer center, where you're basically going from soup to nuts," I replied. "You're starting with the basic biology and then taking that into the clinic. Exploring it all."

Paul and I agreed that such a facility would broaden our understanding of the cellular and molecular mechanisms of aging. We could fully explore how aging affects cancer all the way from preclinical trials to clinical trials, and tailor therapy for patients, according to age. Paul was definitely on the same page, and I left that second visit to Baltimore feeling like I couldn't work anywhere else but Hopkins.

In early 2019, I announced that I was leaving Wistar, but I was sad to leave a place that meant so much to me. I was very close to my colleagues, and retain close ties with many, so leaving was emotionally challenging on multiple levels. Happily, six of the seven people in my lab there decided to go with me to Hopkins, which is somewhat uncommon in the sciences. They'd been through so much with me, exploring aging's crucial role in cancer, and they wanted to continue to do so in my Hopkins lab. They knew, as well as I did, that we were on to something big, and we were determined to pursue it, together.

Soon after my return to Hopkins, I began to recruit additional cancer and aging researchers as part of my commitment to making my vision of a center a reality. To make it truly come together, I had to move beyond only ideas, and beyond the realities of forming its physical space. What I ultimately had to do was to bring together important groups from across the Hopkins campus to approach our research bolstered by the strengths of collaboration. As I write this, I'm finishing a proposal that aims to pull together programs that have anything to do with aging and cancer at Hopkins. These would include the Bloomberg School of Public Health, the School of Medicine, Biomedical Engineering at Homewood—the list continues to swell, because when you bring in different technologies, different disciplines, different perspectives, your chances at finding real solutions becomes much more likely. The promise of connecting so many great minds, paired with the resources and will to follow through on the most promising ideas, is truly thrilling. Who knows what breakthroughs lie around the corner?

Yes, we've returned to my belief in the power of collaboration—how such cooperation and teamwork can change our world for the better. There is an old Swahili saying: to go fast, go alone; to go far, go together. And from what I've seen of cancer, how well I've gotten to know it over my decades of study, I'm certain that such an approach is our only way forward to conquering it, or at the very least, taming it.

A CRITICAL PIECE OF THE PROCESS

The size of my laboratory, on the third floor of Johns Hopkins University's Bloomberg School of Public Health, might surprise you. At two thousand square feet, the lab is as large as a fair-sized house, with plenty of space for a living room, dining room, kitchen, family room, and bedrooms. Of course, our workspace is allotted much differently. But I offer those dimensions to give you an idea of this place, my second home.

The building we're in is a rectangle with a hole in the center. The windows in the lab face inward, so we have a glorious view of the central heating unit and brick walls. The equipment ranges from cabinets full of flasks for experiments to a vegetable steamer lying on the counter that we use as part of a process to stain tissues attached to a slide.

Under fluorescent lighting, there are six rows of benches, making up 12 workstations. Each bench has equipment for a specific technique such as a Western blot bench, a bacterial techniques bench, an imaging bench, and so on. At the end of each bench are desks where people keep their personal belongings and papers and do their computer work.

Along one side of this giant room stands a row of freezers,

where we keep our supplies and reagents. Just across the hall is our tissue culture room, where we do anything related to cell work. We also have a large liquid nitrogen freezer and a microscope, with four sterile flow hoods that resemble medium-sized deli cases.

The complete roster for my lab is 12 people, including postdoctoral fellows, a PhD student, an assistant professor, a research associate, and a lab manager. While everyone has particular assignments, there's plenty of overlap, and I urge people to reach out to each other. If something isn't tracking or making sense for you, if it doesn't seem right, look around and bring one of your colleagues into the conversation; their perspectives and ideas will teach you much more than you can ever learn when operating in a silo. I have only a few guidelines for my lab staff: "Check Your Ego at the Door," "No Divas Allowed," and "Teamwork Makes the Dream Work." That's the key, I believe, when it comes to successfully investigating cancer, and to the smooth operation of a lab. It comes down to the quality of the data and documentation, and how honest and detailed our conversations and collaborations can be.

One of the strangest, most fascinating, and utterly essential processes in our laboratory is making artificial skin. It's a vital tool in our melanoma research efforts and is a prime example of a series of groundbreaking collaborations that have paid immense dividends in multiple spheres of medical research. The story of how tissue engineering came about underscores what we can accomplish when we don't let barriers and biases stop us from working with people from different fields. It also reflects how scientists routinely rely on the researchers who came before them, and build on their progress.

In the 1970s, a pediatric orthopedic surgeon at Boston Children's Hospital named W. T. Green conducted experiments in an effort to create cartilage. While his effort didn't succeed, some of his conclusions led to understanding how, once biocompatible materials were invented, cells could be seeded onto scaffolds.[1] Around the same time, John Burke, a surgeon with a background in chemical engineering (then with the Shriners Burn Institute in Boston) reached out to Ioannis Yannas, an assistant professor of materials science at the Massachusetts Institute of Technology. They collaborated over more than a decade on laboratory and burn patient studies to introduce Silastic in 1981—the first commercially reproducible engineered "neodermis" connective synthetic skin—using a collagen-chondroitin matrix (borne from cow tendons and shark cartilage) to support the growth of dermal fibroblasts to bridge damaged to healthy skin. The flexible, regenerated skin protected patients from infection and dehydration—and wasn't rejected by immune systems.[2] The next generation of their invention, now known as Integra, is still relieving misery and saving lives today.

In 1984, Robert Langer, a chemical engineer at MIT, and Joseph "Jay" Vacanti, a surgeon at Harvard Medical School, wanted to address the shortage of organs available for life-saving transplants. Their goal was to grow new tissues and even new organs in the lab. One of their first projects was developing functional tissue equivalents; to do so, they designed scaffolding built from branching networks of biocompatible and biodegradable polymers for cell delivery that was engineered specifically for this purpose, rather than using something that exists naturally. From these and other early experiments and successes, the field and business of tissue engineering expanded globally.

A former colleague of mine at Wistar, Meenhard Herlyn, optimized this technique for melanoma research purposes, and we learned the procedure from him. Since then, we've used it extensively, but whenever anyone asks, "Can we have your protocol for making artificial skin?" I'll say to them, "I'm happy to give it to you. But I recommend that you send a student to my lab, too, who can learn it in person." It's a tricky process that takes about eighteen days.

Today, many of the cells used in growing artificial skin for cancer research come from neonatal foreskins, which are removed during circumcisions and then donated to research. One foreskin can yield enough cells to make four acres of grafting material for artificial skin because it grows so quickly (the average sample size of a piece in the lab isn't very big, just a couple of centimeters in diameter at most). These fibroblasts are formed on mesh scaffolding by combining molecules of lactic acid and glycolic acid. You're essentially trying to trick extracted fibroblasts into believing that they're still in the human body. If so, they'll communicate with each other to create new skin.

While there's certainly plenty of science involved in the process, a little luck can come in handy, too. Not every batch of artificial skin, no matter how well the instructions are followed, will grow as we need it to. The joke in our lab is that to ensure success you need to stand on one leg, even hop around at bit, when completing crucial stages. Gloria Marino is an American Latina scientist in my lab (and a PhD candidate in the Bloomberg School of Public Health—I'm her thesis advisor) who has experience growing the skin, especially for the extracellular matrices or ECMs. These fill the spaces between cells and help bind the cells and tissue together. Here's how she describes the process:

> If you're making a piece of artificial skin, you start with keratinocytes and feed them cell food, then add different growth supplements as it starts to build up. The skin grows in a stack, a little thicker every day. Once it gets thick enough, you expose the top layer to air and then, if things go well, the cells will secrete what they need to keep growing. When you look at it under the microscope, it resembles a tiny rock formation. You're building these layers, one after another, by adding the growth supplements and exposing it to the air. But like many processes

in science, it can be finicky. You follow the directions and then get to the end and something may have gone wrong. Making a centimeter-sized piece of skin? It's all a little subjective.

As Gloria knows, there's nothing worse than making a batch of artificial skin that can't be used. You've been waiting for about three weeks, and then you're forced back to square one. The good news is that once we have a quality batch, we can use it for multiple experiments. We'll embed it in paraffin or store it in sterile containers or freeze a good batch until it's needed. The engineered skin holds up for a long time—we're still using slices from batches that we made eight years ago.

A pediatric surgeon, a chemical engineer, a surgeon specializing in burn victims, a material sciences professor, a melanoma researcher—and many other scientists—all led to our having this invaluable tool in my lab at Johns Hopkins that the next generation of students are now learning from. This is only one example of a discovery and application sequence that reflects multiple generations of multidisciplinary scientists working hand in hand toward life-saving solutions.

It's a good lesson. In our lab at Hopkins, work begins at about eight in the morning, with everyone arriving by 10:30 a.m. There's a running joke that most of us have such predictable hours that you could set up something like a train schedule for us. Usually, there are seven to ten people working at any given time, a relatively small team, with the emphasis, again, on collaboration and including lots of areas where there's expertise overlap—gears working together. No one's reluctant to ask for help, to bring someone else in if they're puzzled or stymied by something. Having everyone hunkered down in their own private settings doesn't pay off in the long run. That's sometimes a concern that I have about our efforts nationally. Cancer doesn't care who gets credited for supposedly solving a certain component of the disease and who might have a new insight on another. As we've seen, it will rapidly and methodically attack the body once it has an opening. We cannot let our egos get in the way of that basic understanding. We'd miss so many opportunities if we didn't seek out the contributions of others, to see where multiple ways of looking at a problem, and synergies from our respective successes, could lead us.

GETTING THE JOB DONE

One of the characteristics that makes Johns Hopkins a globally recognized university and research center is that the people here, campus-wide, just want to get the science done and move the research forward to solutions. Despite having so many of the top-level experts, including in the cancer field, it's highly collaborative and generally free of the frustrations of parading egos.

Added to this mission-driven approach is a welcome measure of warmth and collegiality. I refer to my fellow chairs in the Bloomberg School of Public Health as my "Band of Chairs." There isn't an issue or question that I'm reluctant to bring to their attention; the atmosphere offers complete confidence to ask anything. All of this made the transition back to Hopkins a pleasant and invigorating experience.

When I returned, we initiated a series of exciting new studies. Of course, the COVID-19 pandemic slowed our progress. We were out of the lab for several months, and when we came back, we were at just 50 percent capacity. While that's been frustrating, we're still forging ahead, and Mitchell Fane, an Australian scientist in the lab, is at the forefront of a new study that is currently in revision for a major journal. His work is uncovering exciting new directions for us in understanding metastasis.

> When I joined the lab, Ashi was really looking at how the primary tumor can get into the bloodstream and move to other organs. That's one of the main things we wanted to ask together: What happens when tumor cells move away and begin to metastasize elsewhere? Melanoma, no matter where its site of origin, can metastasize to the brain, the kidneys, the liver, the lungs. We wanted to know what's happening once the cancer gets to all these sites. What we've found is pretty amazing and it emphasizes the difference in those fibroblasts, the construction workers of the skin, in younger and older patients. One of the interesting

things we've found is that when the melanoma cells get into these different organs, they tend to *not* grow at first. They often go into dormancy, and this protects them from the immune system. When they're dormant, it's harder for the immune system to recognize and eliminate them.

The aging immune system is something that fascinates both Stephen Douglass and Alexis Carey in my lab. Stephen is interested in how the immune system in the local microenvironment changes in conjunction with secreted factors such as Wnts, and also with aging. His work has shown that Wnt5A is secreted by myeloid cells and may be a driver of T-cell exhaustion, which is a phenomenon we also see in aging.[3] Alexis is a PhD candidate in my lab, and she's working on a fascinating project spurred by her deep interest in bone marrow. She's trying to understand how changes in aging bone marrow might educate the primary tumor and cause changes in the immune microenvironment therein.

Laura Heuser is a German postdoc whose start in the lab was interrupted by COVID. Her first day was supposed to be the day after the United States shut its borders to all European flights. When restrictions lifted and she got here, she hit the ground running, and is looking at those "bubbles" we talked about earlier, the exosomes (p. 21), and how the messages they carry when released from cells and traveling through the body change with age.

Another promising project in our lab involves how melanoma cells can escape therapy by using glutamine or fats. In such cases, fatty acid uptake and subsequent fatty acid oxidation helps the tumor cells not only survive but metastasize. In a study published in the September 2020 issue of *Cancer Discovery*, my talented postdoc Gretchen Alicea and I explored how aged fibroblasts increased the secretion of neutral lipids, especially ceramides, which are a family of waxy molecules.[4] We found that the melanoma cells take up lipids from the aged fibroblasts, through FATP2, a fatty acid transport protein; that can allow them to resist targeted therapy. Gretchen is from Puerto Rico and her creative approaches reaffirm how adding in the diversity of culture can expand the diversity of scientific thought.

With this particular study about lipid metabolism and FATP2, age played a pivotal role. We saw that the FATP2 transporters were elevated in the melanoma cells grown in aged skin. It was elevated in tumors that were implanted in younger mice, and it was elevated specifically in the tumors of aged mice. Such understandings about how the body works will help us with further studies. As Gretchen, who led our investigation, says,

> For too long, age has been an afterthought when it comes to treatment. It's traditionally a factor or consideration that occurs closer to the end of clinical trials—when

results are being categorized. Our study demonstrated that the age of the patient is critical to our understanding. The difference in our bodies, between young and older patients, is so important. We need to take that into account early on, for any trial or treatment. That way we can better identify the changes in the body and come up with better treatments that are specific for older patients, especially for melanoma.

And there are other parameters to think about too—it's not just age. We're excited about new data comparing results across age and sex as well. We're investigating the role skin fibroblasts play in young versus aged males, as well as how that compares with young versus aged females. There are striking differences in metabolism between young males and young females, as well as differences in the levels of senescence.

Some of these differences in gender were not unexpected given the previous clinical data. Yet what's interesting is we're beginning to see that in women, the probability of cancer steadily climbs with age, whereas in men, it's logarithmic. By that I mean the rates can jump, sometimes dramatically, in men. Yash Chhabra in the lab, yet another immigrant scientist—twice over, in fact, having immigrated from India to Australia, then Australia to here—has found that this is reflected at the cellular level, where cells also show major differences in metabolism, as well as changes in cell survival pathways and differences between male and female fibro-blasts, which are the cells responsible for making the extra-cellular matrix and collagen. These differences between men and women surprised us and are opening up new streams of exploration.

Focusing on the science. Getting the job done. That was our goal during the COVID-19 pandemic. Through it all, such work will make cancer far less inevitable in the long run. When I consider what we were able to do during such challenging times, how we found a way to continue our work in spite of the practical obstacles and the impacts of the virus on everyone, I'm excited by what we'll discover in the near future now that we're operating at 100 percent capacity again.

CHAPTER 5

Reducing Cancer Diagnoses and Mortality

OUR BODIES ARE GENETICALLY PROGRAMMED to work with all the parts collaborating. In many ways, it reminds me of the thousands of doctors working worldwide to solve the riddle of cancer. When things are functioning, everything inside us comes together, pulling in the same direction. Our normal cells are equipped with regulatory mechanisms that in many cases "can correct damage, abort the process, or even cause hopelessly wrecked cells to destroy themselves," as Mark Wolverton wrote in *Wired*.[1]

Yet, as we all know and as we've seen in our lab, the system becomes more prone to fail us as we grow older. Somewhere a vital protein is being altered or destroyed, and that mutated cell divides to create another; as the process outpaces the growth of normal cells, this disease becomes a dangerous reality for another person. As we grow older, internal natural selection will begin to favor the cancer mutations, and then they may break away and metastasize elsewhere in the body.

At first glance, cancer appears to move in lockstep with

aging. The chances of our getting it, in some form, rise as life expectancies go up around the world. We all know people who've combatted it until they couldn't fight anymore. Still, when we begin to look beyond the raw numbers and textbook definitions for cancer, we can glimpse a different world with more optimistic and hopeful outcomes. We may never cure cancer, at least not all of its many types. Still, it's clear that we're doing a better job of understanding this disease and moving toward ever new ways to keep it at bay and battle it successfully when it crosses the threshold.

Things aren't always as they appear to be. We've heard that a million times in our lifetimes, and it even holds true with how cancer cells appear under the microscope in the lab. Take a look at a normal monocyte cell. With its long, treelike dendritic branches, it's likely one of the creepiest things you've ever seen. But these monocytes help the body fight infections and viruses. They are a basic component of any vibrant immune system.

A melanoma cell, on the other hand? While melanoma cells are dangerous and invasive, they don't appear to be anything special at first glance. They're mostly round, maybe a bit oblong at times. Seemingly nothing to worry about, right? Yet they represent a rule of cancer research: Appearances can be deceiving.

If things aren't necessarily as they appear that can be a cause for hope, too, especially if we're able to change or alter a few key variables. Elsewhere in the body, other cells serve as sentry guards or traffic cops. These are dendritic cells, and they can alert T cells, the body's so-called foot soldiers, to attack the tumors. Yet, as we age, these sentries and soldiers can weaken, and now the tumor cells are better able to do their work unchecked.

Identifying and helping key cells and systems is one way forward in terms of therapy. We recently published a paper that details how blood vessels growing in normal cells are dictated by a specific protein.[2] As we age, we lose that protein and another protein takes over. Until recently, the cancer drugs we had developed only targeted the first protein, which did older patients little or no good at all. Now we're focusing on the role of that second protein. Such instances emphasize why we need to be specific about age and what age groups people fall into. In the case I just mentioned, if you're under 45, the drug works, at least to some extent. But if you're over 45 it doesn't, because the very protein that you're trying to target doesn't exist in the body anymore. We're doing more studies with the emphasis on older patients. Such research has been largely overlooked in the past; that's no longer the case in labs like ours.

Also, we need to keep in mind that cancer treatment and care can differ greatly from what we've found in other chronic diseases, such as heart disease or diabetes, where patients can be given bypass surgery, stents, or statins. Surgeons fix heart valves mechanically. If the operation is successful, it's done and the patient moves on with their life. That's not usually the case with many forms of cancer, although sometimes a tumor can be surgically removed before it metastasizes, and chemotherapy or other treatments can give that patient many additional years with their families.

Our understanding of cancer is changing quickly, and with it our ability to manage and even control the disease. And that's being borne out across many forms it may take—whether breast cancer, lung cancer, melanoma, or other types. The odds of our being able to manage it continue to increase. That's where the advances in immunotherapy are so promising. We need to remember that often only a few cells and how they react and respond to therapy can make all the difference. If we can gain a bit more insight and understanding about these pivotal cells, we'll be even more able to successfully target them for treatment.

Our immune system is divided into two categories.[3] The dendritic cells, the traffic cops, belong to the innate immune division. Others here include the mast cells, which produce histamines to attack allergens, the neutrophils, which kill bacteria, forming pus, and last, but certainly not least, we have the macrophages, with long tendrils to better snag their targets. This type of white blood cell is named after the Greek words for "big eaters."

The innate system needs to work in concert with the adaptive system, which includes B cells and T cells. Both of these are formed in the bone marrow and work hard to keep the cancer cells in check. How well one's immune system works is determined largely by heredity. It comes down to the cells you were born with, whether you had a mother who had breast cancer, for example, or another relative with a different form of cancer. In such cases, cancer borders upon an inevitable diagnoses because of the major role genetics can play—but mortality is not necessarily inevitable. The advances in breast cancer detection and treatment are a perfect example of this, with many more women surviving for years and even decades after their diagnoses.

Cancers that are behaviorally driven are clearly not inevitable. If you smoke, we know that can lead to lung cancer. If you're prone to spend a lot of time in the sun, that can lead to skin cancer. With these and other forms that are avoidable, including those connected to obesity, it's about education, getting the word out; when that happens, the diagnosis and death factors can be lowered exponentially.

Also, we need to further embrace the power of early detection—and make it accessible (financially and geographically) to more people. Screening procedures, some of which were put in place decades ago, have proved to be effective in reducing the worst impacts of cancer by catching it in earlier stages. This applies to genetically, behaviorally, and even some environmentally driven cancers.

Thankfully, the science is improving every day. New trials are held, new research studies are published, new drugs are approved. So, if we don't want cancer to be inevitable, we need to stay educated on the latest advances, and understand how it affects myriad populations in unique ways—young, old, male, female, Black, Hispanic, Asian, white. That goes for everyone in the health care community—from the doctors to the patients.

What makes cancer different from other chronic diseases is that if a few cancer cells escape detection or treatment, the disease will likely return. That's been a given for a long time, and some may find this frightening. To me, though, it's one of the most intriguing things about cancer—what makes it such a puzzle. For example, studies indicate that if tumors leave the primary site early in their life, they can travel to the distant sites, and they may then just sit there, dormant and in wait. As we age different changes can drive these tumors out of dormancy—can make them grow and present with metastasis. If we can better understand how and why these cancer cells are moving about, talking with other cells, the role that age can play, cancer becomes less inevitable. With our research, we're defining the factors that are in play and beginning to determine how everything fits together.

CONSIDERATIONS TO KEEP IN MIND

Don't sunbathe.
Don't smoke.
Don't eat bad stuff.
Exercise.

Those are my basic guidelines for dealing with what I call environmental "insults"—the behavioral side of cancer prevention. At first, this may sound like the do's and don'ts that your mother once told you—something like wearing your coat when it's cold or slipping on your galoshes when it rains. I want to emphasize that I'm not scolding or shaking a finger at anyone here. That said, if we can each take more responsibility for our basic health, it can greatly help our efforts against cancer.

People may not realize that when they smoke or lie in the sun at the beach (or work outside for a living), they're damaging normal cells and driving their transformation to cancer cells at that particular moment. Indeed, these insults drive a chronic accumulation of genetic damage that builds up over time. When this is linked with the immune system's increasing inefficiency as we age, it opens the door to any number of problems. Over time, the microenvironment can become "the ideal soil for the abnormal cancer seed," wrote Azra Raza, author of *The First Cell*.[4]

We're finding that some of this genetic damage has been incurred early on, before the age of 20.[5] The cells are accumulating mutations and it's not just the cells that ultimately become melanoma cells. It's also the normal cells that surround those melanoma cells, and the breakdown of these normal cells can grow over time. Some cells may be genetically reprogrammed to become a melanoma tumor and can grow and metastasize.

Obviously, we know that the body changes as we grow

older. We begin to have gray hair or we may have a bit more trouble moving around. Such factors can serve as a reminder that we need to monitor things—really look out for ourselves on a number of levels. The American Cancer Society recommends that men and women, ages 50 years and older, meet with their health care providers and be regularly tested: men for colon, prostate, and lung cancer; women for breast, cervical, colon, and lung cancer.

In the lab, we're reminded that one's lifestyle can be so important, too. Obesity is emerging as a risk factor with multiple types of cancer (including liver, thyroid, breast, ovarian, pancreatic, stomach, colon, and kidney cancers), and, again, age is a key factor, perhaps in an unexpected way. A 2019 study funded jointly by the American Cancer Society and the National Cancer Institute found that six of 12 obesity-related cancers increased in successive generations of adults ages 25 to 49.[6] Lack of physical activity and greater consumption of calorie-dense fast foods were cited in the study. "Due to the obesity epidemic over the past 40 years, younger generations worldwide are experiencing an earlier and longer-lasting exposure to excess adiposity over their lifetime than previous generations," the researchers wrote. It's thought this may be linked to the alarming increase in the rates of colon cancer in younger patients.

I was recently talking with a colleague who's studying how increasing one's fiber intake, adding a few more vegetables and whole grains to the daily diet, can make a world of difference, too. She's finding these small measures to be important in the treatments she's doing for melanoma. After upping their fiber intake, her patients were seeing better test results and response to therapy within a few weeks.[7]

It's best to avoid fast foods, highly processed meats, and sugary drinks as much as possible. Those fall into my category of "bad stuff." In comparison, whole grains, citrus fruits, and vegetables (carrots, garlic, and onions) have proved to be effective cancer-fighting foods. Longitudinal studies have also indicated that people who exclude meat completely from their diet have far fewer cancer diagnoses.[8] Vegans in these studies had the lowest rates of cancer. It isn't only the direct plant-based food benefits (including higher levels of fiber) driving the findings, though; vegans and vegetarians are also less likely to be overweight, which further reduces their risks.

The link between tanning and cancer, of course, is much better established. With that in mind, I'd urge everyone to use sunscreen (a sun protection factor [SPF] of 30 or above) and wear a wide-brimmed hat when they're outside. Most skin cancers are caused by too much exposure to ultraviolet rays. Their strength depends upon several factors, including time of day (they're at their strongest during mid-day), time of year (stronger in the spring and summer), and altitude (stronger at higher elevations). Also, keep in mind that UV rays are present even on cloudy days. A sunscreen that has an SPF of 15 can filter out about 93 percent of ultraviolet rays, according to the American Cancer Society. In comparison, a SPF sunscreen of 30 eliminates nearly 97 percent. Still, remember that no sunscreen offers complete protection, and none are waterproof.

In our lab, we're investigating the effect UV rays can have as we age. Asurayya Worrede, who came with me to Johns Hopkins from Wistar in Philadelphia, is directing a new study in which we're analyzing the differences as well as the similarities between UV-induced proteins and skin cells. We take cells from punch biopsies of the skin, usually in the upper arm because that hasn't been as exposed to the sun over time as much as the face and other areas of the body. We have several dozen people in various groups—men and women, ages 25 to 35, and men and women, ages 55 to 65.

In the lab, we have a machine that appears to be nothing more than a black box. Yet with this machine, a UV irradiator, we can control the dosage level, as well as the type of the UV rays to which we expose our experimental cells. UV rays are divided into three major categories— UVA, UVB, and UVC. For this study, such differences aren't a major factor. Thankfully, we don't have to worry about UVC rays in our everyday lives as the ozone layer shields us from most of their impact. It's UVA and UVB that age and wrinkle skin cells, and they can damage the cells' DNA, too. Of the two, UVB has slightly more energy.

In another study, we've been varying the doses of UV as we explore how these rays can impact younger patients. For example, does such damage build up over time? And if so, how does that occur? In addition, we're radiating samples of skin of older people. Can such cells, even after years of exposure, take a turn for the worse? "The great thing about our lab is the range of questions being asked," Asurayya says. "They can be in-depth and far-reaching. There's really no limit at all."

When it comes to smoking, no form of tobacco is deemed safe today. Also, it's important to avoid second-hand smoke as much as you can, as that can lead to several forms of cancer. A recent study by the American Heart Association discovered that people who quit smoking cigarettes before age 40 lessen their chances of premature death from cardiovascular disease by 90 percent.[9] The study tracked nearly 400,000 people for 17 years and found that smokers were three times more likely than nonsmokers to die of heart disease or stroke.

In recent years, our understanding of exercise, how important it is, has grown, too. The American Cancer Society recommends that most adults should strive for 150 minutes to 300 minutes of moderate physical activity a week.[10] It can be difficult to begin a new exercise plan on your own, so partner up with a friend. Catch up with each other during a brisk walk. With moderate exercise, you should be able to talk while doing so. After you've gotten started, you can increase the heart rate in future weeks and months.

Yes, we've probably heard much of this advice before. Still, the new studies and the work in our lab and from other places

Protecting Yourself and Your Family

Each of us can help better our odds by being more vigilant about our health. Annual checkups and screenings could save you or your loved one's life, and they should be part of your health care plan. Early detection is one of the most vital tools in the fight against cancer, as self-examinations and scans help technicians and doctors reveal telltale indicators in time to fight them successfully with surgeries and treatments. But, many don't go for these screenings, even though many health insurance plans cover these tests and visits completely as part of their wellness efforts. A survey in 2020 by *Consumer Reports* found that 52 percent of Americans say they never go to the doctor to have their skin checked.[1] Reversing that trend alone would improve melanoma survival rates and save thousands of lives each year.

For skin, breast, cervical, prostate, lung, and colon cancers, annual screenings are recommended by the age of 50. At such appointments, be sure to discuss your family's medical history, asking relatives beforehand if necessary. While some cancers are harder to detect, pay attention to your body through self-examinations as well as noting symptoms that seem out of the ordinary. Jot down any symptoms or discoveries you've made regarding spots, lumps, coughs, pains, or other potentially problematic physical signs before your visit; having a written list will help you remember to tell your doctor each unusual thing you've noticed.

If you have a family history of cancers like melanoma (grandparents, parents, siblings), have recently had cancer yourself, or have more than fifty moles over your body, you may need to see a dermatologist or other specialist more frequently than every 12 months. There's peace of mind in being checked head to toe by a dermatologist using a dermatoscope, with its magnifying lens and pinpoint lighting, and by technicians using the latest equipment and software during mammograms, biomarker lung cancer screenings, and colonoscopies.[2] Researchers and inventors are also focused on new methods that can reveal cancer in early stages, including a blood test that detects more than fifty forms of cancer with 99.3 percent specificity, some before symptoms appear, based on a recent trial with nearly 7,000 participants.[3]

Even if you've been a sunbather, smoker, or have other habits or genetics that could lead to cancer, it need not be a certainty that you will get it or succumb to it if it's diagnosed. Begin conversations with your family doctor now to explore how you can work together to put the brakes on detectable cancers.

Notes

1. Wadyka S. July 9, 2020. How to spot skin cancer. *Consumer Reports*. https://www.consumerreports.org/cancer/how-to-spot-skin-cancer/.

2. Mayo Clinic. *Patient Care and Health Information, Tests and Procedures: Lung Cancer Screening.* https://www.mayoclinic.org/tests-procedures/lung-cancer-screening/about/pac-20385024.

3. Landsdowne LA. July 14, 2020. Blood detects over 50 different cancers with a 0.7% false-positive rate. *Technology Networks*. https://www.technologynetworks.com/cancer-research/blog/blood-test-detects-over-50-different-cancers-with-a-07-false-positive-rate-337305; Liu MC, Oxnard GR, Klein EA, Swanton C, and Seiden MV. June 1, 2020. Sensitive and specific multi-cancer detection and localization using methylation signatures in cell-free DNA. *Annals of Oncology* 31 no. 6: P745–P759. https://www.annalsofoncology.org/article/S0923-7534(20)36058-0/pdf; Blood test detects over 50 types of cancer, some before symptoms appear. *ScienceDaily*, March 30, 2020. https://www.sciencedaily.com/releases/2020/03/200330203241.htm.

are a steady reminder about how important such daily measures can be. Take care of yourself. When we all follow the science (in addition to using our common sense), it makes cancer less inevitable.

ADVANCES IN IMMUNOTHERAPY

Immunotherapy or immune-cell therapy uses the body's immune system to move against cancer. This approach describes a wide range of treatments, and it holds so much promise, especially with melanoma, because it targets specific mutations in a person's cancer. Steven Rosenberg, chief of surgery at the National Cancer Institute, told the *Wall Street Journal* that immunotherapy is the new "blueprint" in therapy.[11]

While immunotherapy is not used as widely as chemotherapy, surgery, or radiation therapy as of yet, it's on the rise (sometimes in combination with those other therapies), and it's one of the most widely used forms of therapy in treating melanoma. In the last few years, we've seen a number of advances within immunotherapy, including T-cell transfer therapy, monoclonal antibodies, immune system modulators, and immune checkpoint inhibitors. Jim Allison is widely recognized for having discovered immune checkpoints and applied them to cancer therapy,[12] and for this he won the Nobel Prize in 2018 along with Tasuku Honjo. Checkpoints are mechanisms by which immune cells are regulated, such that when an immune response is mounted, it doesn't flare out of control and attack cells in the body indiscriminately. However, cancer cells co-opt these mechanisms, and use checkpoints to inhibit the immune response to the tumor cell, such that the tumor can escape from attack and clearance by immune cells. Blocking checkpoint proteins, therefore, is proving to be especially effective in treating melanoma, and we achieve this by using antibodies against immune checkpoint proteins, to essentially bind them up and stop them from triggering an initiation of a checkpoint. These new drugs release the natural brakes on the immune system, allowing them to really go after the cancer. By blocking checkpoints, we can free the T cells and other immune system foot soldiers to move against the cancer.

Some newer advances in understanding the way the immune system works in cancer include the discovery of a T-cell co-stimulatory signal. This is nicknamed "the gas pedal," as it can heighten the T-cell activity. It's one thing to release the brakes within the immune system, to allow the T cells to attack the cancer. It's quite another to accelerate the process, to make it more effective by speeding things up. This gas pedal/brake analogy has long been used to describe oncogene activation in cancer—an oncogene is a mutated form of a gene (known as the wild type) that drives abnormal cell growth. This can lead to the growth of cancer cells. Mutations in genes that become oncogenes can be inherited or caused by being exposed to substances, those behavioral insults, in the environment.[13]

What's wild is that so much else can also impact the immune microenvironment and response to therapy. We see that older patients actually do much better on immune checkpoint therapy. Why? It could be the high mutational burden in these tumors, or the differences in immunomodulatory signals. My friend Jen Wargo at MD Anderson is showing that the microbiome of the gut can also affect patient response to immunotherapy, further feeding the hypothesis that diet and exercise can help provide a better outcome.[14] Already we're seeing such insights and changes in therapy extend to the patients. It used to be that you had to go in for an IV procedure for such treatments to be effective. It was done as an outpatient, going to the hospital, doing the entire procedure there. Increasingly, patients are able to do much of their treatment at home, in pill or capsule form, and are even being provided with "meals to go" in clinical trials to manipulate microbiota. Also, we're becoming better able to monitor progress by various types of scans and blood work. Such tests can measure the size of the tumor and any changes in the blood work.

As a result of such new procedures, we're seeing a growing group of cancer patients who are living longer. Not that long ago, Stage IV melanoma was typically fatal within a year. Today, we're seeing more of these patients live years longer, some even eventually being declared cancer-free. A famous example is former president Jimmy Carter, who was diagnosed with melanoma that eventually spread to the brain. He was treated with checkpoint inhibitors, and several years later, continues to thrive, building houses for Habitat for Humanity, and generally benefiting society through his kind and generous actions, and the work of The Carter Center.

By using the power of the immune system, we're transforming this field of medical care. Today, roughly half of the people diagnosed with advanced melanoma have become so-called super survivors. One of them is my friend T. J. Sharpe. A Stage IV melanoma patient, T. J. was diagnosed in August 2012 with melanoma tumors in multiple organs, only weeks after his second child was born. Since then, he has undergone six surgeries and four immunotherapy treatments and has been involved in two landmark clinical trials. He's chronicled his journey on a blog and in a YouTube video:

> When I was 37, I went into the ER with what I thought was a spiking fever and left 16 days later with a Stage IV melanoma diagnosis. The oncologist who admitted me gave me my tumor report. And when my wife Jen asked him what we were looking at, he said, "I'll be surprised if he's here in two years."
>
> So, after I was diagnosed, I had a lot of time for research, sitting in the hospital for two weeks, to determine what my next steps were. I knew that it wasn't going to be just a regular standard of care, I had a two-month-old son. I didn't want him to grow up without a father, and I was determined to find the best treatment.
>
> It was discouraging realizing I had so few options,

until I started understanding the clinical trials that had different drugs that weren't available to the general public. After realizing that clinical trials were likely my best option, we began looking at every available trial for a Stage IV melanoma patient.

We decided to get several second opinions and found a cancer center that offered a unique trial, and one that I became the first patient ever to get a series of therapies in a certain order. That to me was going to give me the best chance to watch my children grow up.[15]

T. J. empowered himself. He studied what he was up against, networked like crazy, and enrolled in a suitable clinical trial. Incredibly, he ended up receiving much of his treatment only a short drive from his home in Florida. He's not only an example of how proactive a patient sometimes needs to be, but, more importantly, he's an example of the promise that these new rounds of treatment for melanoma may hold for a growing number of people.

LOOKING TO THE FUTURE

We've refined drug treatments so that patients are living five to ten years longer. With nearly a quarter of those patients, specifically those with melanoma, we're using the word "cure." Things are moving at breakneck speed, which gives those of us in cancer research confidence and reason for optimism. And it's not just in melanoma research. The work with breast cancer is advancing rapidly, and in colon cancer, too. Even in pancreatic cancer, advances are being made.

We've also begun to witness that the work being done in one field, say melanoma, can be extrapolated to other forms of cancer. Even a few years ago, we weren't sure that such an effect or trend could happen. But now we're learning about one form of cancer and seeing how that can drive other cancers. For example, Dan Zabransky is an oncology fellow whom I co-mentor with the brilliant Liz Jaffee, deputy director of the Sidney Kimmel Comprehensive Cancer Center at Hopkins, and a pancreatic cancer expert. Dan is extrapolating our aging data in melanoma to pancreatic cancer, under Liz's tutelage. The way immunotherapy is working in melanoma is being studied by researchers dealing with other forms of cancer, such as pancreatic cancer in Liz's lab, breast cancer, and colon cancer—the finding that a particular mutation in colon cancer could sensitize colon cancer cells to immunotherapy was made right here at Hopkins, by Luis Diaz, in collaboration with the Vogelstein/Kinzler lab.[16] In addition, many labs in cancer research are working on various vaccines, which could help with different forms of the disease.

As I look ahead, I'm hopeful because we're beginning to better understand the conversations between the tumor and the stromal cells and the immune cells. We're beginning to understand how to interrupt those conversations when they become harmful to the body—how to block one from the other, how to stop the conversation and make the immune system more active when it needs to be.

The science is speeding ahead, and, in recent years, it's been accompanied by a better sense of cooperation and collaboration. I find this as encouraging as any particular study. Unlike 10 or 15 years ago, you're now fully encouraged to submit collaborative grants. The National Cancer Institute advises hospitals and research centers to do this, and the truth is to get a quality paper published these days you need to work together. There's so much that goes into it that no single lab can possibly do everything all the time. For example, the genomics and sequencing need to be verified and studied in cells and animal experiments. Not all of that is going to be one person's, one place's expertise, so you collaborate with others to do the best work.

Look at many of the papers being published today. They often have 20 to 25 authors, and they're composed of data from three, four, or five different labs. We've learned that you can't do quality science with everyone in their own silos, refusing to work with others. We'll never cure cancer that way.

If you had told me a decade ago that 20 to 30 percent of melanoma patients—even some with Stage IV melanoma—would be in remission for five to ten years, I wouldn't have believed it. Even now, it borders on the miraculous to me. But that's where we are, on the threshold of this new world of research and care.

It's an exciting place to be. Sometimes, when it comes to the new discoveries and how much our understanding grows day by day, it's a real race to keep up. Yet then I wonder about what we're going to learn and better understand come tomorrow, and I cannot wait to see what's next.

Sometimes I think back to when I was a student, decades ago now, and I was peering through the microscope at what the cells in those petri dish "swamps" were doing, captivated by their movement, their interactions. This sense of wonder and fascination has never left me. It drives me every single day toward the answers.

My infatuation with science has brought me halfway around the world, from Lesotho to Maryland to Philadelphia, and eventually to my lab at Hopkins, where I work with some of the most talented and supportive people I've ever known. Our back and forth, our very conversations in the lab, have become as detailed and as dynamic as what goes on moment to moment between the cells in our bodies. Given the political climate we've lived through during these last four years, we have had a lot of cause to think about the power of words, and the impact of hate speech. In a way that's how I think about the conversations that drive malignancy. We're listening and learning, testing and questioning, and ultimately discovering how to interrupt the malignant conversations when we can, and determining how this disease, which has been documented since ancient Egypt and the pharaohs, can become less and less inevitable for all of us.

Acknowledgments

ONE NEVER HAS SUFFICIENT SPACE on an acknowledgments page to thank all of the individuals who have guided their career. First and foremost, I want to thank the extraordinary trainees and collaborators who have graced my professional life—our trainees often teach us more than we teach them, and without them, none of the research in this book would have been performed. My collaborators are based not only at Hopkins, but are spread all over the world, and they make the work fun and add fascinating layers to it. They are my mentors, my role models, and most importantly, my friends. Some who have been instrumental are mentioned in the book, but each one has contributed so much along the way.

Being a scientist is a demanding job and often takes time away from family. I'd like to dedicate this book to my incredible and supportive husband, Pat Morin, and my brilliant and amazing daughter, Alina. They always understand when I'm tied to my computer or on calls at inconvenient times, and when I am free, they're always there to provide me with love and laughter. Pat even patiently read each page of this book and provided helpful comments.

I want to thank my immense support network—from my

patient and loving friends to my family: my mother, brother and sister, whom I mention in this book, and my wonderful niece Tara and nephew Sean, and their little families. Also my adopted family, the Sengamalays, who have been here all along when my parents and siblings were oceans away. Without their love and support I would be nowhere, and their love for me and pride in me gives me confidence when I need it most.

This book would not have happened without my coming to Johns Hopkins in the first place—for that I'd like to thank Denis Wirtz, who was beyond persistent and has been a staunch ally and supporter all the way. I'd also like to thank Arturo Casadevall and Dean Ellen Mackenzie, who opened my eyes to the immense possibilities at the Bloomberg School of Public Health, Bob Casero for orchestrating that connection, and Bill Nelson, Landon King, Liz Jaffee and others at the Cancer Center for partnering so closely with Ellen, Arturo, and Denis to recruit me here.

A huge thank you goes to Tim Wendel, author of *Cancer Crossings*, for his superlative writing skills. In the craziness of my day-to-day schedule, the weekly hours spent chatting with Tim were relaxing and fun. Also, Anna Marlis Burgard provided so much guidance, and her editing skills were critical in making this book easier to understand. Thanks also to Matt McAdam for his helpful comments and to the awesome Julie Messersmith in the Office of Research for supporting this series, and for all she does for us BDPs. And, thanks to

Barbara Kline Pope, publisher and director of Johns Hopkins University Press; this series is her brainchild.

I want to acknowledge the millions of patients and survivors of cancer worldwide, and the tireless patient advocates and foundation staff members who are instrumental in driving funding initiatives, and telling us, the basic scientists, what's most important as we delve into the intricacies of this disease. Their passion fuels ours and makes our science stronger.

Notes

PREFACE

1. Simon S. January 8, 2020. Facts & figures: 2020 reports largest one-year drop in cancer mortality. American Cancer Society. https://www.cancer.org/latest-news/facts-and-figures-2020.html.

2. World Cancer Research Fund/American Institute for Cancer Research, Worldwide Cancer Data: Global cancer statistics for the most common cancers. https://www.wcrf.org/dietandcancer/cancer-trends/worldwide-cancer-data.

CHAPTER 1. THE NATURE OF CANCER

1. American Cancer Society. [undated]. Early history of cancer. https://www.cancer.org/cancer/cancer-basics/history-of-cancer/what-is-cancer.html.

2. Ling Y, Zhou QZ, Situ HL. Study on therapy of breast cancer by Chinese traditional medicine. In Li SL, ed. *Human Breast Tumor*, 537–549. Beijing: Scientific and Technical Documentation Press 2000.

3. Tsoucalas G, Karamanou M, Laios K, Androutsos G. 2019. Rhazes' (864–925) views on cancer and the introduction of chemotherapy. *Journal of the Balkan Union of Oncology* (JBUON) 24(2): 868–871.

4. Akhikairi S. November 20, 2019. Top 10 epidemic diseases that were common in the ancient world. *Ancient History Lists*. https://www.ancienthistorylists.com/ancient-civilizations/top-10-epidemic-diseases-that-were-common-in-ancient-world/.

5. Pott P. 1775. *Chirurgical observations relative to the cataract, the polypus of the nose and cancer of the scrotum*. London: T. J. Carnegy.

6. Boveri T. 1902. *Über mehrpolige Mitosen als Mittel zur Analyse des Zellkerns* [Concerning multipolar mitoses as a means of analyzing the cell nucleus]. *Verh. d. phys. med. Ges. zu Würzburg* NF, Bd. 35. See also Boveri T. 2008. Concerning the origin of malignant tumours. *Journal of Cell Science* 121:1–84. doi:10.1242/jcs.025742.

7. Lane-Claypon JE. 1926. A further report on cancer of the breast with special reference to its associated antecedent conditions. *Reports on Public Health and Medical Subjects,* no. 32.

8. Mukherjee S. 2010. *The Emperor of All Maladies: A Biography of Cancer,* 43–45. New York: Scribner.

9. Population Reference Bureau. December 1, 2002. Americans are living longer than ever. https://www.prb.org/americansarelivinglongerthanever/.

10. Vincent G, Velkoff V. May 2010. Current population reports: The next four decades. US Census Bureau, US Department of Commerce.

11. American Cancer Society. [2021]. Survival rates for melanoma skin cancer. https://www.cancer.org/cancer/melanoma-skin-cancer/detection-diagnosis -staging/survival-rates-for-melanoma-skin-cancer-by-stage.html.

12. American Cancer Society. 2021. Cancer facts and figures. https://www. cancer.org/research/cancer-facts-statistics/all-cancer-facts-figures /cancer-facts-figures-2021.html.

13. Swerdlow J. January 2017. Unmasking skin. *National Geographic,* 122–123. https://www.nationalgeographic.com/science/article/unmasking-skinb. See also Institute for Quality and Efficiency in Health Care (IQWiG). September 28, 2009, updated April 11, 2019. How does skin work? https:// www.ncbi.nlm.nih.gov/books/NBK279255/.

14. Cancer.Net. March 2018. Stages of cancer. https://www.cancer.net/ navigating-cancer-care/diagnosing-cancer/stages-cancer.

15. Paget S. 1889. The distribution of secondary growths in cancer of the breast. *The Lancet* 133 (3421): 571–573.

16. Alicea GM, Rebecca VW, Goldman AR, Fane ME, Douglass SM, Behera R, Webster MR, Kugel CH III, Ecker BL, Caino MC, Kossenkov AV, Tang HY, Frederick DT, Flaherty KT, Xu X, Liu Q, Gabrilovich DI, Herlyn M, Blair

IA, Schug ZT, Speicher DW, Weeraratna AT. September 2020. Changes
in aged fibroblast lipid metabolism induce age-dependent melanoma cell
resistance to targeted therapy via the fatty acid transporter FATP2. *Cancer
Discovery* 10 (9): 1282–1295. doi: 10.1158/2159-8290.CD-20-0329.

CHAPTER 2. THE ROLE OF CANCER RESEARCH

1. Soto SM. 2013. Role of efflux pumps in the antibiotic resistance of bacteria
   embedded in a biofilm. *Virulence* 4 (3): 223–229. doi:10.4161/viru.23724.

2. Mukherjee S. 2010. *The Emperor of All Maladies: A Biography of Cancer*,
   122–127. New York: Scribner.

3. Wendel T. 2018. *Cancer Crossings: A Brother, His Doctors and the Quest
   for a Cure to Childhood Leukemia*, 108–109, 115–117. Ithaca, NY: Cornell
   University Press.

4. Wendel, *Cancer Crossings*, 40.

5. Wendel, *Cancer Crossings*, 8.

6. Baker SJ, Fearon ER, Nigro JM, Hamilton SR, Preisinger AC, Jessup JM,
   vanTuinen P, Ledbetter DH, Barker DF, Nakamura Y, White R, Vogelstein
   B. April 14, 1989. Chromosome 17 deletions and p53 gene mutations in
   colorectal carcinomas. *Science* 244 (4901): 217–221. doi: 10.1126/science
   .2649981.

7. Weeraratna AT, Jiang Y, Hostetter G, Rosenblatt K, Duray P, Bittner M,
   Trent JM. April 2002. Wnt5a signaling directly affects cell motility and
   invasion of metastatic melanoma. *Cancer Cell* 1 (3): 279–288. doi: 10.1016
   /s1535-6108(02)00045-4.

8. Bittner M, Meltzer P, Chen Y, Jiang Y, Seftor E, Hendrix M, Radmacher
   M, Simon R, Yakhini Z, Ben-Dor A, Sampas N, Dougherty E, Wang E,
   Marincola F, Gooden C, Lueders J, Glatfelter A, Pollock P, Carpten J,
   Gillanders E, Leja D, Dietrich K, Beaudry C, Berens M, Alberts D, Sondak
   V. August 3, 2000. Molecular classification of cutaneous malignant
   melanoma by gene expression profiling. *Nature* 406 (6795): 536–540. doi:
   10.1038/35020115.

9. Morin PJ, Sparks AB, Korinek V, Barker N, Clevers H, Vogelstein B, Kinzler

KW. Activation of beta-catenin-Tcf signaling in colon cancer by mutations in beta-catenin or APC. March 21, 1997. *Science* 275 (5307): 1787–1790. doi: 10.1126/science.275.5307.1787.

10. Weeraratna et al., Wnt5a signaling.

11. Moon RT, Campbell RM, Christian JL, McGrew LL, Shih J, Fraser S. 1993. Xwnt-5A: a maternal Wnt that affects morphogenetic movements after overexpression in embryos of Xenopus laevis. *Development* 119 (1): 97–111.

12. Weeraratna et al., Wnt5a signaling.

13. Velarde MC, Demaria M, Campisi J. January 17, 2013. Senescent cells and their secretory phenotype as targets for cancer therapy. *Interdisciplinary Topics in Gerontology* 38: 17–27. doi: 10.1159/000343572.

CHAPTER 3. BREAKING THROUGH

1. Morin PJ. 2007. Claudin proteins in ovarian cancer. *Disease Markers* 23 (5–6): 453–457. doi: 10.1155/2007/674058.

2. Zahn JM, Poosala S, Owen AB, Ingram DK, Lustig A, Carter A, et al. 2007. AGEMAP: A gene expression database for aging in mice. *PLoS Genet* 3(11): e201.

3. Bissell M. June 2012. Experiments that point to a new understanding of cancer. TED Talk, https://www.ted.com/talks/mina_bissell_experiments_that_point_to_a_new_understanding_of_cancer?language=en.

4. Kaur A, Webster MR, Marchbank K, Behera R, Ndoye A, Kugel CH 3rd, Dang VM, Appleton J, O'Connell MP, Cheng P, Valiga AA, Morissette R, McDonnell NB, Ferrucci L, Kossenkov AV, Meeth K, Tang HY, Yin X, Wood WH III, Lehrmann E, Becker KG, Flaherty KT, Frederick DT, Wargo JA, Cooper ZA, Tetzlaff MT, Hudgens C, Aird KM, Zhang R, Xu X, Liu Q, Bartlett E, Karakousis G, Eroglu Z, Lo RS, Chan M, Menzies AM, Long GV, Johnson DB, Sosman J, Schilling B, Schadendorf D, Speicher DW, Bosenberg M, Ribas A, Weeraratna AT. 2016. sFRP2 in the aged microenvironment drives melanoma metastasis and therapy resistance. *Nature* 532: 250–254. https://doi.org/10.1038/nature17392.

5. Krtolica A, Parrinello S, Lockett S, Desprez PY, and Campisi J. October

2001. Senescent fibroblasts promote epithelial cell growth and tumor-igenesis: a link between cancer and aging. Proceedings of the National Academy of Sciences 98 (21): 12072–77. doi: 10.1073/pnas.211053698.

6. Campisi J, d'Adda di Fagagna F. 2007. Cellular senescence: When bad things happen to good cells. *Nature Reviews Molecular Cell Biology* 8: 729–740. https://doi.org/10.1038/nrm2233.

7. Kugel CH III, Douglass SM, Webster MR, Kaur A, Liu Q, Yin X, Weiss SA, Darvishian F, Al-Rohil RN, Ndoye A, Behera R, Alicea GM, Ecker BL, Fane M, Allegrezza MJ, Svoronos N, Kumar V, Wang DY, Somasundaram R, Hu-Lieskovan S, Ozgun A, Herlyn M, Conejo-Garcia JR, Gabrilovich D, Stone EL, Nowicki TS, Sosman J, Rai R, Carlino MS, Long GV, Marais R, Ribas A, Eroglu Z, Davies MA, Schilling B, Schadendorf D, Xu W, Amaravadi RK, Menzies AM, McQuade JL, Johnson DB, Osman I, Weeraratna AT. 2018. Age correlates with response to Anti-PD1, reflecting age-related differences in intratumoral effector and regulatory T-cell populations. *Clinical Cancer Research* 24 (21): 5347–5356. doi: 10.1158/1078-0432.CCR-18-1116.

8. Jain V, Hwang WT, Venigalla S, Nead KT, Lukens JN, Mitchell TC, and Shabason JE. 2020. Association of age with efficacy of immunotherapy in metastatic melanoma. *Oncologist* 25 (2) e381–e385. doi: 10.1634/theoncologist.2019-0377.

9. Sceneay J, Goreczny GJ, Wilson K, Morrow S, DeCristo MJ, Ubellacker JM, Qin Y, Laszewski T, Stover DG, Barrera V, Hutchinson JN, Freedman RA, Mittendorf EA, McAllister SS. Interferon signaling is diminished with age and is associated with immune checkpoint blockade efficacy in triple-negative breast cancer. *Cancer Discovery* 9 (9): 1208–1227. doi: 10.1158/2159-8290.CD-18-1454.

10. Morin P, Wirtz D, Weeraratna A. September 14, 2020. Completing the great unfinished symphony of cancer together: The importance of immigrants to cancer research. *Cancer Cell* 38 (3): 301–305. https://www.sciencedirect.com/science/article/abs/pii/S1535610820304281.

CHAPTER 4. A VISION FOR FUTURE CARE

1. Vacanti CA. 2006. The history of tissue engineering. *Journal of Cellular and Molecular Medicine* 10 (3): 569–576. doi: 10.1111/j.1582-4934.2006.tb00421.x.

2. Burke JF, Yannas IV, Quinby WC Jr, Bondoc CC, Jung WK. October 1981. Successful use of a physiologically acceptable artificial skin in the treatment of extensive burn injury. *Annals of Surgery* 194 (4): 413–428. doi:10.1097/00000658-198110000-00005.

3. Douglass SM, Fane ME, Sanseviero E, Ecker BL, Kugel CH III, Behera R, Kumar V, Tcyganov EN, Yin X, Liu Q, Chhabra Y, Alicea GM, Kuruvilla R, Gabrilovich DI, Weeraratna AT. February 2021. Myeloid-derived suppressor cells are a major source of Wnt5A in the melanoma microenvironment and depend on Wnt5A for full suppressive activity. *Cancer Research* 81 (3): 658–670. doi: 10.1158/0008-5472.CAN-20-1238.

4. Alicea GM, Rebecca VW, Goldman AR, Fane ME, Douglass SM, Behera R, Webster MR, Kugel CH 3rd, Ecker BL, Caino MC, Kossenkov AV, Tang HY, Frederick DT, Flaherty KT, Xu X, Liu Q, Gabrilovich DI, Herlyn M, Blair IA, Schug ZT, Speicher DW, Weeraratna AT. September 2020. Changes in aged fibroblast lipid metabolism induce age-dependent melanoma cell resistance to targeted therapy via the fatty acid transporter FATP2. *Cancer Discovery* 10 (9): 1282–1295. doi: 10.1158/2159-8290.CD-20-0329.

CHAPTER 5. REDUCING CANCER DIAGNOSES AND MORTALITY

1. Wolverton M. May 5, 2013. "The way we think about cancer must evolve," *Wired*.

2. Fane ME, Ecker BL, Kaur A, Marino GE, Alicea GM, Douglass SM, Chhabra Y, Webster MR, Marshall A, Colling R, Espinosa O, Coupe N, Maroo N, Campo L, Middleton MR, Corrie P, Xu X, Karakousis GC, Weeraratna AT. November 2020. sFRP2 supersedes VEGF as an age-related driver of angiogenesis in melanoma, affecting response to anti-VEGF therapy in older patients. *Clinical Cancer Research* 26 (21): 5709–5719. doi: 10.1158/1078-0432.CCR-20-0446.

3. Institute for Quality and Efficiency in Health Care (IQWiG). 2006 (updated July 30, 2020). *The Innate and Adaptive Immune Systems.* https://www.ncbi.nlm.nih.gov/books/NBK279396.

4. Raza A. 2019. *The First Cell and the Human Costs of Pursuing Cancer to the Last*, 81. New York: Basic Books.

5. Thomas H. Mutation and clonal selection in the ageing oesophagus. *Nature Reviews Gastroenterology Hepatology* 16 (2019): 139. https://doi.org/10.1038/s41575-019-0117-y.

6. Bath C. April 25, 2019. Rising rates of six obesity-related cancers among young adults. *ASCO Post.*

7. Wargo JA. September 11, 2020. Modulating gut microbes. *Science* 369 (6509): 1302–1303. doi: 10.1126/science.abc3965.

8. Mayo Clinic Staff. October 20, 2019. How plant-based food helps fight cancer. Mayo Clinic. https://www.mayoclinic.org/healthy-lifestyle/nutrition-and-healthy-eating/in-depth/how-plant-based-food-helps-fight-cancer/art-20457590.

9. Searing L. January 18, 2021. If you smoke, quitting before age 40 could dramatically lessen your chances of an early heart-related death. *Washington Post.*

10. American Cancer Society. June 9, 2020. American Cancer Society guidelines for diet and physical activity. https://www.cancer.org/healthy/eat-healthy-get-active/acs-guidelines-nutrition-physical-activity-cancer-prevention/guidelines.html.

11. Burton TM. October 12, 2017. Immunotherapy treatments for cancer gain momentum. *Wall Street Journal.*

12. Gillenwater B. October 4, 2018. James Allison: The main act. Rockville, MD: National Foundation for Cancer Research. https://www.nfcr.org/blog/szent-gyorgyi-prize-allison-immunotherapy?gclid=CjoKCQiAhP2BBhD-dARIsAJEzXlH6HXLF1M45tGe2nzegTWALZOWFO-6SPjPkKNiSOK73ZI-HOMHelPoQaAqzMEALw_wcB.

13. National Cancer Institute. Immunotherapy to treat cancer. https://www.cancer.gov/about-cancer/treatment/types/immunotherapy.

14. Wargo JA. September 11, 2020. Modulating gut microbes. *Science* 369 (6509): 1302–1303. doi: 10.1126/science.abc3965.

15. Sharpe TJ. April 4–5, 2018. Keynote Presentation: Bridging clinical research and clinical health care. National Harbor, Maryland. https://www.youtube.com/watch?v=pc2i6hJceio.

16. Le DT, Durham JN, Smith KN, Wang H, Bartlett BR, Aulakh LK, Lu S, Kemberling H, Wilt C, Luber BS, Wong F, Azad NS, Rucki AA, Laheru D, Donehower R, Zaheer A, Fisher GA, Crocenzi TS, Lee JJ, Greten TF, Duffy AG, Ciombor KK, Eyring AD, Lam BH, Joe A, Kang SP, Holdhoff M, Danilova L, Cope L, Meyer C, Zhou S, Goldberg RM, Armstrong DK, Bever KM, Fader AN, Taube J, Housseau F, Spetzler D, Xiao N, Pardoll DM, Papadopoulos N, Kinzler KW, Eshleman JR, Vogelstein B, Anders RA, Diaz LA Jr. July 28, 2017. Mismatch repair deficiency predicts response of solid tumors to PD-1 blockade. *Science* 357 (6349): 409–413. doi: 10.1126/science.aan6733. See also Le DT, Uram JN, Wang H, Bartlett BR, Kemberling H, Eyring AD, Skora AD, Luber BS, Azad NS, Laheru D, Biedrzycki B, Donehower RC, Zaheer A, Fisher GA, Crocenzi TS, Lee JJ, Duffy SM, Goldberg RM, de la Chapelle A, Koshiji M, Bhaijee F, Huebner T, Hruban RH, Wood LD, Cuka N, Pardoll DM, Papadopoulos N, Kinzler KW, Zhou S, Cornish TC, Taube JM, Anders RA, Eshleman JR, Vogelstein B, Diaz LA Jr. June 25, 2015. PD-1 blockade in tumors with mismatch-repair deficiency. *New England Journal of Medicine* 372 (26): 2509–2520. doi: 10.1056/NEJMoa1500596.

Index

MORE IN THE WAVELENGTHS SERIES

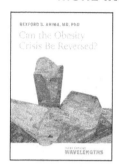
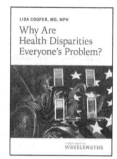
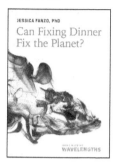

Can the Obesity Crisis Be Reversed?

Rexford S. Ahima, MD, PhD

"Dr. Ahima's experience shines through in this update on treatment approaches and helpful strategies for those dealing with the chronic disease of obesity."—Kelly Allison, Director, Center for Weight and Eating Disorders, University of Pennsylvania

Why Are Health Disparities Everyone's Problem?

Lisa Cooper, MD, MPH

"Dr. Cooper's personal and professional journey is both riveting and inspiring. *Why Are Health Disparities Everyone's Problem?* is not only an essential read but a central question for our time."—Marc H. Morial, President/CEO, National Urban League / former Mayor of New Orleans

Can Fixing Dinner Fix the Planet?

Jessica Fanzo, PhD

"Jessica Fanzo has seen it all, read everything, and talked to everyone. You can have no better, more knowledgeable guide to the mess the food system is in, and how we can get out of it. If you want to do something about the global nutrition crisis, read her book, and roll up your sleeves, as she does."
—Luigi Guarino, Crop Trust / Svalbard Seed Vault

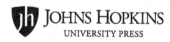

press.jhu.edu